Understanding
the Adolescent

Understanding
the Adolescent

George H. Orvin, M.D.

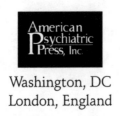

American Psychiatric Press, Inc.

Washington, DC
London, England

Copyright © 1995 American Psychiatric Press, Inc.
ALL RIGHTS RESERVED
Manufactured in the United States of America on acid-free paper
98 97 96 95   4 3 2 1
First Edition

American Psychiatric Press, Inc.
1400 K Street, N.W., Washington, DC   20005

Library of Congress Cataloging-in-Publication Data
Orvin, George H., 1922-
    Understanding the adolescent / George H. Orvin.
        p.   cm.
    Includes bibliographical references (p.   ) and index.
    ISBN 0-88048-651-1
    1. Adolescence.   2. Adolescent psychology.   3. Parent and
teenager.   4. Teenagers—Family relationships.   I. Title.
HQ796.O674   1995
305.23′5—dc20   95-24033
                                                                        CIP

British Library Cataloguing in Publication Data
A CIP record is available from the British Library.

Contents

~~~~~~

Dedication   vii

Introduction   ix

Section I
Adolescents, Families, and Parents

~~~~~~

1 Family Environment and Its Effect on Children   3

2 Adolescents and Their Parents   25

3 Communicating With Adolescents   37

4 Setting Limits for Adolescents   53

Section II
Who Are Adolescents?

~~~~~~

5 Normality and Adolescence   73

6 Adolescents' Evolving Personal Identity   93

7 Adolescents' Evolving Sexual Identity   105

Section III
Problems in Adolescence

8 Adolescents' Risk-Taking Behavior 125

9 Serious Problems That Occur in Adolescence 139

Section IV
Late Adolescence

10 Transition Into Adulthood 163

Conclusion 177

References 181

Index 183

Dedication

~~~~~~

One of the benefits that comes from writing a book is the privilege of writing a dedication. I dedicate this book to many people because many people made it possible. My thanks begin with my parents, Jesse W. and Ruth Walton Orvin. They not only made the book possible; they made the author possible. And they provided me with a happy childhood, a happy home, and two wonderful role models. They gave me a brother, John W. Orvin, and three sisters, Miriam O. House, Anne O. Yarborough, and Shirley O. Munn, who contributed to the enrichment of our family life.

I thank my teachers for their perseverance and their endurance in providing me with a good education.

I thank the many adolescents and their parents who came to my hospital and taught me how to understand them and how to help them as they struggled to manage their lives.

I thank the many bright and energetic professionals who helped me organize and operate a specialized environment in which dysfunctional adolescents and their families could be healed. I thank the many trainees who came to learn and then went into the world to further the healing of so many others. I thank my colleague, R. Layton McCurdy, M.D., for his encouragement and years of professional support.

I thank my children: Candace Palmer, Jay Scott Orvin, Debra Ann Orvin, and Nancy Lee Ward. So much of my learning came from them. I thank them for perceiving my love. And I thank them for growing up to be healthy, productive, and likable people. Much of the credit for that goes to their mother.

For their mother, I am grateful to her dear parents, G. Clifton and May Stewart Salvo. And I am grateful to her elderly cousins, Sallie and John Arnold, for their loving adoration of her.

Thus, I have thanked the "many" who have contributed to this book. But most of all, I thank my wife. I thank her for her constant love, her forbearance, her gentleness, and her undiluted womanhood. I thank her for mothering our children and helping me become a father, and then helping me to be a father. But most of all, I thank her for being my wife and helping me to be a husband. I thank her for helping me become what I have become.

Now, all of the effort that has gone into this book becomes fulfilled as I dedicate it to my wife, Rosalie Salvo Orvin.

Introduction

~~~~~~

"What am I going to do with my 13-year-old?" Here is a question that transcends all boundaries of race, religion, or cultural circumstances and is near and dear to the hearts of parents worldwide; if there is one thing more difficult than being an adolescent, it is having one. This isn't a "how to" book; most parents already know how to raise their adolescent. But the "how to" can become easier if parents can understand the processes of development and the interplay of those processes one on the other. If parents can understand what is happening to their adolescent, they might endure their adolescent's thrashing about better.

Although adolescents face major challenges in their movement toward adulthood, their parents also face challenges—their own as well as their child's. Everyone seems to try hard to understand the adolescent. Who tries to understand parents? The adolescent? Not likely. The public? Also unlikely. The changes that take place during parenthood are no less challenging and no less exciting than the changes that take place during adolescence. The process of adolescence influences the process of parental relationships. And the process of those relationships has a critical role in the development of the adolescent. If parents can understand what is happening to their adolescent, perhaps they can begin to find joy in other relationships and in each other, because the children will be gone, soon. For those who still have a partner, it will be just the two parents left. With or without a partner, it need not be the end.

Adolescent Anxiety and
Its Effects on Others

Most adults are scared of adolescents. Just being within an arm's length of an adolescent unleashes anxiety in adults. Some adults prefer to think of that anxiety as a dislike for adolescents, especially those professionals who choose not to work with them. I recall my own anxiety as I embarked on a career of treating dysfunctional adolescents. That anxiety was suddenly relieved when I discovered a secret that has since stood me in good stead: it was not *my* anxiety that I felt in the presence of an adolescent; it was the *adolescent's* anxiety.

Adolescents are scared, and well they might be. What other period of life is more frightening and anxiety ridden? Adolescents' anxiety and fear are resonated in others just as the high-pitched note of the violin is resonated in a delicate glass, which then shatters. Of course, adolescents don't appear anxious or fearful as they try to hide their feelings from others and even themselves; instead, they try to be "cool." They hide their fears beneath a layer of insouciance. They cannot tolerate the appearance of uncertainty and fear, as it reveals their vulnerable part and suggests not only a failure to obtain the certainty of adulthood but also a fixation at or a return to the uncertainty of childhood. The nonchalance is a mask that hides doubts and fears. This then is the secret, and, as Josselyn (1971) noted, the adolescent is more inclined to put trust in the adult who recognizes the differences between the adolescent and the behavior, and who refuses to strip away that mask or to ridicule what the mask hides.

A vicious cycle ensues when the adults experience the adolescent's fear and anxiety within themselves, misinterpret it as belonging to themselves, and respond in a posture of self-defense. This then escalates the fear and anxiety in the adolescent, who in turn responds in a posture of self-defense. Ironically, the adolescent finds his or her own anxiety and fear coming home but is unable to recognize their origin. It is natural for adults to respond to the hostile (frightened) adolescent defensively, but counterproductive.

Adolescents and Their Families

Before one can fully determine how to best assist adolescents in their struggles, one must understand what strengths and weaknesses adolescents bring to those struggles—characteristics that are developed in the first decade of life within the context of the family.

In Chapter 1, I focus on the adolescent's family, whether this is a single-parent family, dual-parent family, extended family, or stepfamily. Parents, brothers, sisters, and all who reside in the family are enormously significant parts of the adolescent's external environment. Some of adolescents' struggling is a consequence of their reaction to their environment. But adolescents do more than struggle. They hope and they dream. Not only they, but also their parents, their brothers, their sisters, and all those who live within the structure of the family. The adolescent is growing and reacting to both an internal and an external environment. Aspirations, hopes, and dreams are important parts of an internal environment.

The relationship between parents is an integral part of the family structure. If parents are experiencing difficulties in their relationship, it is likely that those difficulties will reverberate through the rest of the family. For the sake of the family, parents must pay as much attention to their own relationship as they do to the relationship they have with their children. Parents must of necessity nourish and nurture their children, whose needs are, for the most part, quite demanding. What are less demanding and less apparent are the needs of each parent. Indeed, many new parents begin to take pride in "putting the children first." It is during the first 4 or 5 years that parenthood reaches its ascendancy, for it is during these years that parents experience what might be described as *total parenthood*. Too frequently, as the role of mother or father grows, the role of husband or wife withers. All of this has implications for the adolescence of children as well as for the development of their parents.

In Chapter 2, I discuss the relationship between parents and their adolescent. Although there are no golden rules for ensuring a successful relationship, I do offer some general guidelines that should be useful in helping both parent and adolescent treat each other with respect, thereby leading to a healthy and caring relationship. However, even those parents blessed with such a relationship will find it being tested as their adolescent struggles for independence and autonomy. A close look at the changing dynamics of parent-adolescent interactions is offered in the hope that it will ease this transition for both adult and child.

In Chapters 3 and 4, I discuss two areas that can be particular trouble spots for parents: communicating with an adolescent and setting limits for the adolescent. Adults find understanding adolescents to be difficult. They become frustrated when adolescents refuse to reveal what is happening to them. But adolescents are going through a difficult and puzzling time; they cannot explain what they do not understand. If adults have some understanding of the process of change in adolescence, it then becomes less necessary for adolescents to try to supply an explanation, but at the same time more likely that they will try. Communicating with an adolescent isn't always easy. There are no set rules for so doing, but there are some things parents need to keep in mind when trying to communicate with adolescents, which are presented in Chapter 3.

In Chapter 4, I address the process of setting limits for children and offer some guidelines for doing so. Most parents know that children need limits established for them as they grow up. These limits not only help protect children, but also give them a sense of safety. It shows them the boundaries that they should not cross, and the boundaries within which they will be safe. But how do parents suddenly reverse this process and begin withdrawing limits as their adolescent strains toward independence?

Adolescence begins the process of relinquishing control of the child by his or her parents. This process scares both adolescents and parents. The success of an adolescent's gradual move toward autonomy depends in part on where his or her parents are in their own process of becoming and how invested they are in maintaining control over their adolescent.

Adolescents do not meet and master their challenges with a smooth and constantly improving set of skills. Their deportment can be obnoxious and irritating. On occasion it can be charming. The struggle is less charming than difficult. Their efforts to take control of their life cause parents to feel a loss of control. Not knowing how it will turn out and fearing the worst, parents can find themselves in pitched battles with their adolescent. It is at such times when it helps to have another adult with whom one can talk and collaborate. These are the times that can be so difficult for single parents!

Adolescents and the Changes They Experience

In Section II of this book, I turn to adolescents themselves and the changes they are going through. These changes are enormous as a child struggles toward adulthood, emancipation, and autonomy. Biological changes of growth and maturation influence psychological and sociological changes of mental and emotional development, and, to some extent, vice versa. Much of what is happening to the adolescent is exciting and pleasing. Some of what is happening is frightening. Much of what is happening is, for the most part, incomprehensible to the adolescent as much as it is to the parents. The entire process becomes comprehensible eventually by adolescents and parents living through it.

As Cameron (1955) taught, each child brings his or her strengths and weaknesses into the process of evolving identity. Those characteristics make that child who he or she is and will help determine how he or she reacts to the environment. Efforts to understand the adolescent will be influenced by many things, but those who would seek that understanding must remember that most adolescents are as bewildered by the changes that are taking place in them as others might be. Even if they understand the tasks of becoming an adolescent, they still might lack the verbal skills to communicate that understanding to others.

Because of the significant changes that are taking place, an adolescent's struggle can be tumultuous, resulting in odd and inconsistent behaviors. Parents see behaviors in their adolescent they have never seen before and wonder, "Is my adolescent normal?" In Chapter 5, I attempt to describe what are viewed as normal adolescent behaviors. However, in this discussion, I emphasize two caveats. First, the only constant in the adolescence process is change. What is normal behavior for a child when he or she is age 13 might be completely outdated by the time that child reaches age 14. Second, because all adolescents differ vastly from one another, there are no so-called normal behaviors. When I use the word *normal,* I am referring to behaviors that are within normal limits.

It would be misleading to suggest that there is a rank order of importance for each of the challenges adolescents must face. It would be incorrect to suggest that there is a sequence of first this one then that. They are linked one to another, each enhancing or complicating the other. For those who would help the adolescent through the process, it helps to understand each challenge and to understand that those challenges might be disguised or hidden in a bewildering array of maladaptive behavior. But for the most part, the adolescent makes these transitions without damage.

In Chapter 6, the development of a personal identity is addressed. Adolescence is a time of deep self-questioning. One of the skills developed during the teenage years is the capacity for abstract reasoning. Adolescents turn this capacity inward and begin to dissect themselves, limb by limb, to determine whether they like what they see. For some, the answer is yes; for others, it is a demoralizing no. Adolescents also compare themselves with their peers, judging whether they are alike or different. This is a time for forming close relationships with peers, often with one especially close friend of the same gender. Through their relationship with the same and opposite gender peers, adolescents begin to formulate in their mind the role of each gender. Adult models also help in this formulation.

However, for adolescents who have not liked what they have found in their self-evaluation, or who have not found themselves to be lovable by family or friends, the turmoil only churns deeper. These young people, desperate for acceptance and love, will turn to alternative groups of people and means for achieving that approval. This can cause further problems, and make the normally difficult adolescent process of growing toward adulthood almost impossible.

For adolescents, the process of becoming an adult is exciting, but in some ways frightening because it leads to becoming responsible for one's own security. Adolescents must surrender the security that parents have always provided and now begin to provide their own security. But it doesn't end there. They must also begin to think about providing security for someone else in addition to themselves. The journey from consumer of security to provider of security is not brief, not smooth, and not always direct. So the adolescent has a vested interest in remaining dependent as well as a desire to become independent. Parents, even under ideal circumstances, have a vested interest in maintaining childhood since that in turn maintains their parenthood. True, children want to grow up, and, true, parents want children to grow up. For the most part, parents come to terms with their changing roles with their children and children with their changing roles with their parents.

Some of the struggles adolescents go through can be attributed to the biological changes they are enduring. In Chapter 7, I address these changes and the adolescent's evolving sexual identity. Although during adolescence, young people develop the ability to become sexually active, at this stage they do not have the emotional or psychological maturity to fully realize the potential of sexual relations. Instead, there is a potential for short-circuiting the value of this type of relationship in exchange for instant gratification, a shortcut into adulthood, and the illusion of physical intimacy. What is missed is the opportunity to develop the appropriate concept of the role sexuality plays in gender identity and in intimate relationships with others. More visible consequences of early adolescent sexual activity are pregnancy and sexually transmitted diseases.

When Things Go Wrong

In Section III, problems other than those that normally occur during adolescence are addressed. In Chapter 8, I discuss how adolescents are almost instinctually drawn toward taking risks. Some risks are constructive and necessary in order to achieve new goals. However, destructive risks have their origin not in a desire to reach new heights, but in a struggle to establish control over one's life through maladaptive means. Most often adolescents who take these risks are crying for help. Eventually, deleterious risk taking can lead to the need for professional mental health counseling. In Chapter 9, I address some of the problems that can develop out of a troubled adolescence and their impact on the family.

Christine Collange (1988), a mother and well-known writer in France, challenged me and a group of my colleagues with several provocative questions. They are questions that cross the minds of many parents. "Why do people want to make us believe, adults as well as the young, that all the problems of adolescents are connected to our behavior as parents? Why are society and the mass media always slanted toward the poor young people who suffer from their poor relations with their parents and never toward the lot of the poor parents who suffer from their poor relationships with their youth?"

Indeed, there does seem to be a bias. Somehow, self-proclaimed experts seem bent on laying all of the blame on the parental doorstep whenever anything goes wrong in the life of the adolescent. But parents unwittingly contribute to that bias. "Where did we go wrong?" is the reflexive response of so many parents in regard to almost any failing their child might experience. Somehow or another, parents are quick to blame themselves. And good parents do so more than the negligent ones. Understanding the adolescent and understanding the adolescent process can be helpful. But why only the adolescent? Why only the adolescent process? Why shouldn't parents also try to understand themselves? Why shouldn't adults try to understand what is happening to them?

During the course of my career, I have come to know many adolescents who were severely dysfunctional. I was inoculated against the belief that all adolescents were doomed through the privilege of having four normal adolescents of my own, and by seeing, in evaluation, the normal children of worried and frightened parents. But perhaps Madame Collange was right in her suspicion that a conspiracy seems to exist, to the effect that somehow or other, whatever goes wrong with children must be the consequence of poor parenting and inept parents. Perhaps we so-called experts create that impression as we seek, search, and research the causes of childhood dysfunction. Unwittingly, we focus on the "lame and the halt" rather than the healthy. Although we professionals contribute to such a belief, we mustn't claim complete responsibility. There is something about the adolescent process that is unnerving to all of those in the fallout area. Even though we no longer believe that all adolescents must go through turbulence, storm, and strife, we who study them come to know the anxiety and fear which even the normal adolescent seems to provoke.

In the final section, Chapter 10, I look at the process of moving from late adolescence into early adulthood. At this stage in life, young people must face three issues: 1) leaving home, 2) developing true intimacy with another person, and 3) making long-term commitments. Once the threshold into adulthood is crossed and one eventually becomes a parent oneself, the whole process of spousehood, parenthood, and dealing with adolescents begins for a new generation.

Adolescents view adulthood as the "promised land" in their journey of growth. But to dwell harmoniously with others and with the environment, they must acquire new skills and new tools. What worked well for them as dependent, vulnerable, and helpless children will not serve them well as an adult. That which sheltered them in their infancy and childhood will no longer be of benefit. Indeed, some of the things that served them so well yesterday might now become encumbrances. The time now comes when valued concepts must be challenged and indeed changed. Some of adolescents' embedded beliefs will surely disable them if not eradicated before their assumption of adult license and adult responsibility. Some of those beliefs were vital to their successful psychological functioning as children. Their needs as children were those of consumers of security. The time now comes when they must begin to provide their own security and ready themselves to provide security for others.

A Personal Bias

I worry about what happens to adolescents during the crucial work of identity formation. Because I am a psychiatrist, I think like one. Let the reader be so warned. It is a potential bias I readily confess. But I also bring other biases. I am a physician, I am a husband, I am a father, and I am a grandparent. I struggle to avoid the excesses of each viewpoint. My view of the process of adolescence might cause me to overvalue the importance of the vulnerability of the psychologic apparatus. On the other hand, so much of the adolescent's successful adaptation to changing environments, internal and external, depends on an intact psychological structure. Even the healthy and resilient adolescent not only must make major adjustments and adaptations to a changing physical body, but also must resolve significant social and psychological conflicts.

Summary

In the end, parents should find encouragement in their adolescents' changes, because their children are becoming what the parents have been, are, and will be. Parents teach their children how to grow based on the way they conduct their lives. Indeed, children are becoming as their parents are becoming, and they are becoming their parents—warts and all!

Eventually, there can be fulfillment in life as each individual comes to terms with who and what he or she has become. It comes with the recognition that each person's life has been unique. Life has been especially blessed when part of that fulfillment derives from one's learning how to care for another. Through this process of caring, people find that fulfillment and teach their children how to live in an intimate relationship with another human being. In so doing, parents learn how to live and, as parents, teach their children how to live.

Adolescents, Families, and Parents

FEIFFER®

I HATED THE WAY
I TURNED OUT..

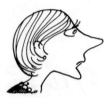

SO EVERYTHING MY MOTHER
DID WITH ME I HAVE TRIED
TO DO THE OPPOSITE WITH
MY JENNIFER.

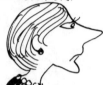

MOTHER WAS
POSSESSIVE. I
ENCOURAGED
INDEPENDENCE.

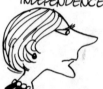

MOTHER WAS MANIPULA-
TIVE. I HAVE BEEN
DIRECT.

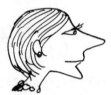

MOTHER WAS
SECRETIVE. I HAVE
BEEN OPEN.

MOTHER WAS EVASIVE.
I HAVE BEEN DE-
CISIVE.

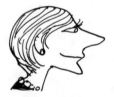

NOW MY WORK
IS DONE. JENNIFER
IS GROWN.

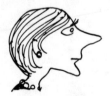

THE EXACT IMAGE
OF MOTHER.

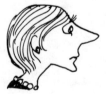

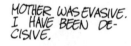

Chapter 1

Family Environment and Its Effect on Children

*T*olstoy (1901) opened *Anna Karenina* with these words: "Happy families are all alike, every unhappy family is unhappy in its own way." It is a safe bet that happy families have a better chance of producing healthy children than do unhappy families. Families come in different shapes, sizes, and states of happiness. To understand what is happening to the adolescent, one must view him or her in the context of the family. Efforts to understand adolescents in isolation from their families fall short of achieving clarity. Even under ideal circumstances, the adolescent is not easily understood.

What Is a Family Today?

The human family is a good bit more than the sum of its parts. It is a living thing with an identity all its own as well as a place of being. It is a system and, as such, has many of the characteristics typical of other systems. It contains subsystems and, at its boundary, touches on other systems, such as educational, occupational, religious, and governmental systems. It touches on other families as well. The *nuclear family* in its ideal form contains a mother, a father, and one or more children. The *extended family* includes grandparents, uncles, aunts, and cousins; it offers social support

3

to supplement and complement the nuclear family.

To suggest that the American family has undergone major changes over the last 10–20 years is to state the obvious. Members of the extended family might now live hundreds of miles away from the nuclear family. Furthermore, the reality of the nuclear family is that it does not always consist of a mother, father, brother, and sister. Divorce, death, and other social changes have altered the shape of the modern family.

In addition, social pressures are having major effects on the integrity of the family system. Poverty, death, drugs, street crime, child abuse, family disruption, and the waning of traditional values of morality are tearing at the fabric of society.

The Role of the Family

The family is a psychological support system designed to sustain its members during periods of adversity. Society needs a steady supply of replacements as death takes its toll. It looks to the family for those replacements and holds the family responsible for transmitting society's values to succeeding generations. Society is structured in a way that it has distinct expectations of families. Society requires a formal contractual agreement between husband and wife not only as a sanction against sexual irresponsibility but also as a means of gaining accountability for the care of any offspring.

Families provide living experiences for children that will help move them from total dependence to independence, from isolation to full integration with their fellow human beings, and from an unformed spirit and personality to fulfillment as an individual, unique in his or her own identity. For better or worse, these experiences help shape our expectation of what our environment will offer us and what it will seek from us as individuals worthy of the respect of our fellow human beings and worthy of the respect of ourselves.

The family—whether a dual-parent family, single-parent family, stepfamily, or family comprising several "extended family" members—has three broad functions:

1. To provide for the physical needs of its members (e.g., food, shelter, protection)
2. To provide for the creation and development of autonomy in children
3. To stabilize and develop the personalities of the parents

Providing for Physical Needs of Family Members

Success or failure in this assignment is fairly easy to determine. This is the easy part when compared with the other two tasks. Adequate food, housing, health care, and safety are critical to the successful functioning of a family and are not easily obtained. Their acquisition is more apparent and less vaguely defined than the other tasks.

Leading Children Toward Autonomy

Once children have been created, how do parents bring about their autonomy while maintaining connectedness? And how does the family participate in the development of their individuality? The family's obligation to its children is to move them toward autonomy, independence, and individuality. Children should be able to leave the family nest and come to stand on their own.

I doubt that parents fully realize their role in facilitating autonomy in their children or, indeed, that they may be thwarting this process. And when this progress toward autonomy is thwarted, most parents do not realize the extent to which how what they are doing can jeopardize an adolescent's development.

As children undertake and attempt to master new tasks, parents can be overly cautious and express doubts about the child's readiness. Not wanting the child to experience disappointment or, perhaps, even harm, parents may discourage children from trying new ventures. On the other hand, understanding the goal of autonomy, parents can and frequently do encourage their children to take on more difficult tasks with "Atta girl," "Atta boy," and "You can do it." It helps to understand the relationship between privilege and responsibility because parents sometimes withhold new responsibilities if they appear to be privileges.

Autonomy can be discouraged by negative attitudes in parents and overly critical comments. Sometimes, growth can be slowed unintentionally by parental caution.

> Lee Ann, a 16-year-old, asked her mother's permission to drive with friends to a nearby beach resort. Ordinarily, her mother would have said "yes," but it was Labor Day, and traffic would be heavy. Her mother would worry the entire time Lee Ann was away, thus spoiling the day for her mother. On the other hand, it would be fun for Lee Ann and would be in the direction of increasing independence. "I won't ask you to stay home although I'll worry until you return. I won't ask you not to go if you won't ask me 'not to worry.'" The deal was struck. Mother gave Lee Ann permission to go, and Lee Ann gave her mother permission to worry.
>
> Sometimes it is much easier to say no than to say yes.

At the same time that parents are teaching their children to pursue autonomy, they must also show them how to value and pursue connectedness with others—that is, to develop their ability to be close to another human being. This pursuit of true intimacy begins within the family but reaches fulfillment beyond adolescence.

Developing Parents' Personalities and the Parents' Relationship

This major assignment for families is too frequently lost in the shuffle.

A rewarding partnership leads to effective parenting.
Marriage marks the beginning of a new relationship for two adults and another opportunity for growth. To the extent that the marriage enhances the growth of each partner, the marriage prospers. To the extent that it prospers, the partners become better prepared for parenthood. Being a parent should enhance the relationship with a spouse or partner but not replace it. A happy and growing wife and husband will make a more effective mother and father.

Parenthood without the true intimacy of spousehood fails to provide the working model of effective caring and loving that is so important for children to see and to feel.

Lewis et al. (1976) described effective marriages as being

> effective in an instrumental sense and charged affectively. Sexuality is gratifying to both; although the frequency of intercourse varies widely from couple to couple, pleasure, gratification, and orgasm are the rule. The husbands are busy and successful, but have energy and affect for their wives and children.

After years of working with dysfunctional families, I concluded that there were many ways parents could disserve their children, but that there was one almost universal failing among these families: the parents did not take care of each other! Parents are in a position to model for their children how human beings live together in an intimate relationship through caring and respect. If parents fail to respect each other, what do their children learn about self-respect?

Parents must take time for themselves. There is a belief that families are mainly for children and that families are where children grow. So heavily committed and invested are some individuals in their parental role that they give little thought, time, or importance to their responsibility to themselves as individuals or to their mates. Many do not understand that, in addition to shaping their children, parents are also shaped by their experiences as they raise their families. Ayn Rand (1961) wrote, in *The Virtue of Selfishness,* that being responsible for ourselves is no vice, and that total selflessness to the extent of never giving unto ourselves is not virtue. How many mothers and fathers present their children with parents who are always tired, unhappy, and deprived?

Parents must care about each other. Perhaps there are many marriages in which the pain is sufficiently manageable that it does not spill over and disrupt the growth of the adolescents. But it certainly disrupts the growth of the parents. No marriages are unending joy, but it seems only fair to expect some joy sometime.

Security comes to children who see their parents caring for each other, and even though the children might test the parental union, they are comforted when the union withstands the test. Ordinarily, children want their parents to be loyal to each other, and they want their family to be firmly intact.

Parents must reevaluate their personal growth. Many of the parents I have come to know seldom take time to contemplate themselves, what is happening to them, and what they should be getting out of all of this struggle. They begin this experience as a young man and a young woman, alone. They complete it as an older man and an older woman, again alone. The time will come when they ask themselves what they have accomplished: "What did you as an individual, and I as an individual, get out of all of this life together, besides these children? What have we learned about each other? Have we grown as individuals, as spouses, and as parents? We have watched our children grow. But did we watch us grow? Together and individually? What sort of people have we become?"

A strong parental relationship encourages autonomy in children. Parents will always maintain a strong role, regardless of what happens to their children, but the more they enshrine parenthood, the more difficult their children will find it to leave them and the more difficult they will find their emancipation and autonomy. The failure to invest in a marital relationship will have serious implications for parents as unfulfilled individuals, but that will not be the only cost. An equally important cost might be borne by their children.

A strong parental relationship builds a flexible atmosphere in which problems can be confronted. When parents invest time in themselves and their relationship, as well as in their children, they go a long way toward providing a setting in which family problems can be readily resolved. Their positive, caring attitudes bring flexibility into the process of living in close proximity with other human beings. It is understandable that such a family setting would give a family its greatest chance for psychological health.

Even healthy families experience stress, and when that stress is severe enough, the family might lose some of its flexibility, at least temporarily.

Changes to Family Structure

Family cohesiveness and effectiveness are affected by the disruptions caused by the loss of a parent through divorce or death, but many families are reconstituted at an effective and functional level. I have had the pleasure of personally and professionally knowing highly effective single parents and stepparents. Although there are some caveats regarding the expectations of newly remarried people, most blended and reconstituted families will work satisfactorily if basic considerations are applied, considerations that are the same as those for the intact family.

Family Changes Following a Divorce

For marriage, the dreaded "D" word is either death or divorce. Those who have experienced the latter suggest that the two experiences are equally painful. When things go wrong for parents, divorce becomes a potential outcome. The advent of adolescence can be the trigger that brings to an end what has been a doomed marriage. But adolescence doesn't cause a good marriage to end! It can only set off unseen forces, which cause disillusioned mates to recognize that a spousehood no longer lives. As the adolescent moves more quickly toward autonomy, the prospect of change can have positive effects on a family, but it can also suggest that the family is beginning to unravel. This is especially so if the adolescent who is about to depart is part of a need-fulfilling relationship with one parent or the other.

Depending on the strength and value of the marital relationship, one parent or the other might begin to feel that life is passing him or her by. If the marriage has not been rewarding, a parent might see the adolescent's unlimited options and freedom in stark contrast to the lack of both for himself or herself. When the marital relationship is valued by both parents, the beginning exodus of children will be endured or, perhaps, even celebrated.

Divorce has an effect on children that can be deleterious. When divorce is a consequence of the undernourished spousehood, at least some damage to the children has already been done. When parents gradually lose the ability or the desire to meet each other's needs, children do not prosper. Even parents who endure each other "for the sake of the children" usually cannot hide the status of their marriage from the children. The rest of the family usually knows that the marriage has ended long before the divorce takes place. I cannot be sure that ending the marriage is worse than continuing it in all of its misery.

The greater damage in a marriage headed toward divorce comes from the ongoing acrimony and vengeance. The parent who is designated the "injured partner" might have the greater difficulty in coming to terms with his or her anger. Therein lies the danger that the "victim" might become more inaccessible to the children than the injuring partner. The damage done to the children of divorce derives less from the fact of divorce and more from the passions that engulf and make the parents unavailable to the children.

Divorce seems a greater tragedy in families with children. Although wounded by divorce, this particular child would not exist if this particular woman and this particular man had not come together to create the child. In some ways, a "bad marriage" might find reason for having existed, if only to produce this particular child or these particular children.

Although a psychological trauma, divorce need not be the end. Out of the disaster of divorce, human growth can occur if there is a genuine search for an understanding of how each person contributed to the problem. Only through such self-questioning is growth possible. Such an endeavor must be more than an attempt to fix blame. Seldom do marriages terminate for a single and simple reason. Rarely can all of the fault be laid at the door of one partner and all of the innocence at the other. As ex-partners learn from the traumatic experience of divorce, they become more responsible for the direction of their life after divorce.

As with other human challenges, ex-partners must utilize the coping skills they have acquired to solve problems they encounter in life. I have seen divorced husbands and wives go on to new relationships and successful marriages with different partners and even with each other. I have seen adolescents work through and come to terms with their anger toward one or both parents. Most children come to understand in adulthood that which they could not understand in their childhood.

Any discussion of divorce should include consideration of life after divorce. Single parenthood poses special challenges for the parent, the children, and the family. Divorce destroys the family that existed prior to the fact. That is, divorce becomes the official recognition of an ending. But the people involved continue to live, although in a different structure of relationships. A new family structure ensues. A single-parent family is considerably different from the two-parent form, but it is still a family.

Single-Parent Families

Most single-parent homes are healthy and productive. Whether the home is led by a single parent because of death of a parent or because of divorce, it does not necessarily follow that it becomes dysfunctional. Children can move toward autonomy and independence despite an absent parent. Indeed, a single-parent home can be more functional and healthier than a dual-parent home if the latter is riven by dissension, distrust, and disloyalty.

However, single parenthood does pose special challenges for the parent, children, and family. The new family structure continues to face all of the challenges of the intact family but carries additional baggage. Financial problems are increased. In addition, the single parent must deal with the complexities of transporting, supervising, disciplining, nourishing, and nurturing the children. Moreover, not only is the load heavier, but it must be borne by the single parent without the collaboration of a spouse. The absent parent represents a loss not only for the children but also for the remaining parent.

It is essential that single parents find psychological support from others. One source of support are groups for single parents, such as Parents Without Partners, which has chapters in most communities. The burdens of single parenthood can also be eased by finding a ready "consultant" in the form of a mate or a very sympathetic and knowledgeable friend. It helps if that "consultant" has walked in the shoes of parenthood. The important thing is that single parents should maintain a connection with others, although this does not necessarily mean that they should remarry.

Sometimes single parents are overwhelmed with advice as to what "should be done." Although self-confidence may be badly shaken by the loss of a mate, most single parents eventually simply do what seems best at the time of the particular event under consideration. That is what all parents must do.

Single parents must also find ways to continue their personal growth without the benefit of a mate. Sometimes the loneliness and fear of the future, which come to all who struggle through life without the benefit of a close and abiding relationship with another adult human being, are the most difficult parts of being a single parent. If the single parent will take time and energy for self-investment, personal growth remains available. It is difficult to be a single parent, but matters are made worse if the single parent commits everything to the task of being a parent and nothing to the task of personal growth.

Stepfamilies

Sometimes the natural course of events for the single parent is the discovery of a new family. Here lies opportunity and here lies danger!

Ordinarily, a family has the luxury of gradual growth. Trust has time to develop. As children are born, children and parents get to know one another slowly and in an environment of mutual respect. Parents learn how to demonstrate their love and have repeated opportunities to earn their child's trust. Children have repeated opportunities to obtain the approval of their loving parents, and they learn how to please those parents. But a reconstituted family does not have the luxury of gradualness. Over a prolonged period, children can and do learn to love, respect, and conform to the wishes of a stepparent. But this process can't and won't happen instantaneously.

"This is your new daddy" or "This is your new mommy" is going to be met with some skepticism, if not outright hostility, by most children, especially adolescents! A new parent may possess many wonderful qualities and might be of great value to children whose family has recently undergone disruption, but if that new parent believes he or she is going to get instantaneous trust and acceptance, he or she is headed for disappointment.

It is absolutely imperative that the parents of a reconstituted family begin their relationship with a clear understanding that the relationship is going to be tested early and frequently. If these new partners do not value spousehood sufficiently, the relationship will end prematurely. If the relationship of the husband and wife in a stepfamily is submitted to the same destructive disaffection that destroyed the previous marriage, they might as well expect the same outcome. It is imperative that they establish clear channels of communication with each other—not only about things but about feelings.

Stepfamilies face great challenges and great opportunities. They urgently need time and understanding. Rivalries are natural between humans, especially siblings. A secret part of the child wants the new marriage to fail. In some ways, he or she wants to go back to the old ways, ways that are perhaps bad but at least familiar. The parents are often burdened with guilt over a failed marriage and fearful of yet another failure; they also need all the help and understanding they can get. Another potential source of trouble in a stepfamily is each parent's tendency to defend, protect, and help his or her own child before all others. This tendency is natural and proper for any parent. But in the context of a stepfamily, each parent must be aware of this tendency and constantly guard against unfair behavior toward stepchildren.

One of the major impediments to success in the reconstituted family arises from the strong motivation of the new parent to avoid being the stereotypical stepparent. Wanting to succeed, stepparents sometimes try too hard and too soon. When the new father or mother attempts to enforce discipline for the stepchild, new families get their first test. Many of the strains in a new family grow out of disciplining. Visher and Visher (1979) pointed out that "discipline works only when the person receiving the discipline cares about the reaction of and the relationship with the person doing the disciplining." In other words, when children know that they have the approval of a loving parent, they will do almost anything within their power to maintain that approval. The stepparent who understands this concept, and who has the ability and willingness to communicate that love and that approval, becomes a highly valued adult for that child. But it takes time. Successful stepparents learn the value of being patient and the value of earning trust.

The stepfamily is a wonderful opportunity and can be an instrument of healing. The new parent can be a great resource for children who have been the victims of a failed family. I have known stepfathers and stepmothers who came to be adored by their stepchildren—eventually.

On the adolescent ward in our hospital, we continually go through the same process of earning acceptance and trust as do stepfamilies. Children who came to live with us were there because our setting was designed to provide them with new living experiences and help them feel better about themselves and their family. There were things that I and my staff could offer those children, many of which were similar to those that can be offered in a healthy stepfamily:

- ✦ New ideas
- ✦ New views of old ideas
- ✦ Predictable adults
- ✦ Expressive and affectionate adults

There is always much we can do to help these adolescents as soon as they move onto the ward, but often they are not ready. We have to wait; we have to be tested and found valid. We have to struggle to try and understand how each of the adolescents in our care views the world and how he or she feels. We have to provide an environment in which the adults understand one another, talk with one another, and care about one another. In this setting, the children in our care interact with us and with one another. Here they learn new ways of living. They grow.

Again, much as happens in a family, these adolescents leave us and get on with their lives. We celebrate their growth and their departure. We measure our success not only by their growth but by ours. With that growth, we are able to achieve a sense of fulfillment.

Optimally Competent Families and Competent Families

Families organize themselves in various ways at least partly depending on the parents' experiences in their own respective family of origin. Over many years, Lewis et al. (1976) studied different types of families, ranging from optimally competent to competent to mid-range dysfunctional to chaotic. In focusing on families of healthy and happy adolescents, they found striking similarities between these families and the ones they called *optimally competent families*. Families determined to be *optimally competent* were those that successfully facilitated the developing autonomy in children and provided a medium in which parental personalities could continue to grow. Lewis (1986, p. 33) further described how these families operated:

> They showed a parental coalition characterized by flexibility, shared power, and considerable psychological intimacy. Together, the parents provide strong effective leadership for the family, but they are not authoritarian, rather they listen to their adolescent child's ideas and feelings and seek, whenever possible, solutions through negotiation.
>
> Communication in healthy families is clear and spontaneous. Family members are highly responsible to each other and take responsibility for individual opinions and actions. All kinds of feelings are clearly expressed and empathy is commonplace. Roles within the families are flexible and differences acceptable. Such families use a wide range of processes by which they deal with novelty, change and stress.

Each family is different in certain ways and will use operational styles similar to and different from those used by other families. The fundamental tasks of a family can be facilitated or hindered by family style or family structure. A family environment can invite and stimulate growth of its members if there is an understanding of that objective by the adults who are responsible for the family's organization and operation. Knowing how to bring about that objective is also important, but first we must know that there is such an objective. Each family will apply its own techniques to accomplish its goals. How the family approaches its tasks will depend upon many factors, not the least of which are the attitudes and personalities of the parents.

Lewis et al.'s work with families demonstrated a variety of ways that families use to organize themselves and to function. Adolescents who have the privilege of growing up in a healthy and optimally competent family are more likely to move through adolescence smoothly. It also follows that these children are more apt to be happy. These are children whose parents feel lucky to have such nice children. By and large, families are pleased with their children but tend to worry that something might go wrong.

In general, most families stumble and struggle toward the goal of raising healthy children without ever getting a clear set of instructions on what is needed or how to bring about a healthy family. What factors bring about healthy families? A look at Lewis et al.'s optimally competent families helps us understand how these families function. From observation of their operation, one might draw inferences as to why they functioned well:

1. These families revealed a structure with a well-defined leadership shared by the parents. In certain areas of family life, the mother was the leader, and in others, it was the father. The roles of each parent were consistent, clear, and mutually agreed upon.
2. Authority existed but authoritarian behavior did not. The power of the parents was shared, and the children understood that the parents were in charge.
3. Although there was a sense of closeness in these families, individuality was permitted and encouraged.
4. All members were allowed to express opinions and ideas, but clarity was demanded. All human feelings were expressed and responded to, with each member accepting responsibility for his or her thoughts and feelings.
5. There was an understanding that each would speak only for himself or herself and not presume to speak for others.
6. Family members respected one another.

These families provide a healthy setting in which the husband and the wife can be more than a father and a mother. Effective families produce growth not only in children but also in parents.

The concept of the optimally competent family is more than an ideal abstraction. However, because these families rarely require counseling, they seldom appear in mental health statistics. I suspect that there are far more of these families than many mental health professionals would predict.

Competent Families

Most families seeking mental health counseling fall somewhat shy of being optimally competent. Both the optimally competent family and the competent family seem to produce healthy children. The difference in these two categories stems from the parental relationship and its degree of satisfaction. My own experience with families confirms this observation.

Less than optimally competent families are distinguished by the unhappiness of one or both parents. These parents raise functional children but fail in the acquisition of intimacy and fulfillment for themselves. In my experience, these parents are unhappy with each other, and each feels uncared for by his or her spouse. Whereas even the most functional families have struggles from time to time, for the most part, there seem to be qualities in the marriage that set a theme for the optimally competent family marked by good spirits and the open expression of affection. On the other hand, whereas less than optimally competent families permit the expression of feeling within the family, it is the parental relationship that is pained. Moreover, there is an unspoken agreement to not talk about that pain. These spouses fulfill parental responsibilities and must be seen as good parents. Their family does the sort of things a good family is expected to do for children. The less than optimally competent family fails in the growth and fulfillment of husband and wife.

Dysfunctional Families

It is not my purpose in this book to analyze severely pathological families but to impart some understanding as to how the average family can comprehend the challenges it faces in helping a child grow into functional adulthood. On the other hand, it helps to understand what it is that dysfunctional families do to produce dysfunctional children who become dysfunctional adults and who, in turn, form dysfunctional families that produce yet other dysfunctional human beings.

It might seem simple to determine the right course in raising a family by simply observing those families that function well, but it does not work that way. Many of the families I saw in my practice were struggling mightily and trying to do the "right" things. For the most part, they were doing about as well as they could, given the circumstances of their lives and the skills they possessed to bring to bear on their problems. The parents were madly treading water with their noses just above the surface. The last thing they needed was "one more wave." These were families in pain. These were parents who loved their children, parents who were doing the best they knew how.

The families who brought their troubled children to me were almost uniformly sad families. They had little fun and little enjoyment of one another, anyone, or anything. For most of these families, there was a pervading sense of despair.

Factors That Can Cause Difficulties for Families

Although many of the families I have seen during my 30 years in practice were in one way or another dysfunctional—not necessarily meaning that a mental illness was present—a wide variety of factors led to the dysfunction of those children or those families. Indeed, no one factor could be singled out. Some of the families had functioned adequately until the first child reached adolescence. Others had malfunctioned from the very beginning. In some ways, these families were different from one another, but for the most part, they were more alike than different.

In reading this section, keep in mind that simplistic explanations for why children become dysfunctional often are flawed.

Parents' attitudes and beliefs.   Parents have a natural tendency to bring attitudes, beliefs, sentiments, and behaviors from their childhood into their relationships with their children. Those beliefs and attitudes are outgrowths of each parent's own childhood development and his or her understanding of how his or her family of origin worked, how he or she grew up in his or her family, and how well he or she discovered his or her maladaptations as he or she continued to grow. These biases affect parents' relationship with each other as well as with their children, as seen in the following example:

> A general and his wife came to see a therapist, with the general's wife having finally convinced him that they needed help, but only after their son Jack, Jr., made a fairly serious suicide attempt. "Jack never has a kind word for Jack, Jr. He's a perfectionist and finds fault with everything young Jack does. He grew up in a military family, and his father could not tolerate the least amount of disorder. I don't know how my mother-in-law tolerated it the way she did. Jack takes good care of us, but he sure is hard to please."
>
> Jack, Sr., replied: "She's right, Doctor. I guess I am a perfectionist. But I was raised to believe that any job worth doing should be done to the best of my ability. Helen grew up in a family that was far more relaxed and fun-loving. Her dad was easy going and more demonstrative than mine was."

The general's approach to life had served him well in college and in his career. He was a graduate of the Academy and the first one in his class to be promoted to general rank.

The two people entered parenthood with differences in "rearing" experiences, each convinced that he or she was raised the "right" way. These differences created problems not only for their son but also for each other.

Genetic risks. How well parents do in establishing the right medium for their children's growth also depends to an extent on the parents' genetic endowment. Each of us brings a loading of genetic risk into this world, and some children enter the world with a kind of fragility that seems to conspire against healthiness and happiness. With enough genetic taint, even an ideal environment will be challenged.

Much of the family environment will be a consequence of attitudes brought by the parents from their own family of origin. Each mother brings with her nurturing skills she learned from her mother and other qualities that might not have been learned but inherited. Similarly, each father brings skills and attitudes. As we observe newborn infants, we learn that some are quieter than others and that some are more active. There is certainly a suggestion that each of us comes into the world with constitutional differences. To the extent that some of our human qualities are not the pure result of our environment, they represent our genetic endowment. I have seen children live in a happy and loving environment and do less well than their siblings even when the parenting for each child was not demonstrably different.

Unhealthy environments.   Even psychotoxic environments have been endured by children who seem to have possessed some sort of "psychological antibodies" that made them immune to all manner of outrages. Unfortunately, these antibodies are few.

Inability to communicate feelings.   Parents who have grown up in families in which feelings were not indulged might find difficulty in expressing feelings within the family they come to lead. Perhaps they are not unfeeling people, but only unexpressive.

In my work with families of adolescents, I noticed certain qualities and characteristics within the families that appeared with an unsettling frequency: family members' inability to express their feelings. So many of these parents believed that if they worked hard enough, their children would become well-adjusted adults. Seldom were these parents negligent in their parental responsibilities. Rarely were these children truly deprived of physical necessities. When neglect did occur, it was more frequently in the sphere of emotional deprivation.

Many of these families were uncomfortable in the open expression of affection—in expressing not only love but also anger, jealousy, fear, or sadness. It was difficult for them to say, "How angry I am!" "How scared I am!" or "How terribly sad I feel." Many of these families had lost significant loved ones but had not allowed themselves the luxury of mourning their dead!

Parents who engage in a need-fulfilling relationship with their children. When parents fail to care for and meet the needs of each other, one deprived parent might reach across the generational boundary and involve herself or himself in a need-fulfilling relationship with one or more of the children. It is this generational boundary that constitutes a gap and a barrier for the two generations. It would be incorrect to suggest that breaching this boundary always leads to incest. It is not incorrect to suggest that incest requires a breaching of the boundary as well as a dysfunctional relationship between parents.

Even though incest does not occur, a need-fulfilling relationship complicates the child's development. Parents who feel unfulfilled as a person, as a spouse, or in their career might cling desperately to their role as a parent, thus pressuring their offspring to remain in the role of a child. Once this child becomes an adolescent, his or her movement toward independence will then be threatened; a child's success in working toward autonomy and toward terminating that need-fulfilling relationship can be devastating for the parent. If an adolescent's independence and autonomy are to be endured by his or her parents, it must not lead to an overwhelming loss of the caregivers' total identity.

Parents who did not develop self-esteem in childhood. Much of parents' sense of personal worth and certainly their perception of being able to be loved originated in their experiences as young children in the care of their parents. As they themselves passed through adolescence, they were either helped or hindered in this process by their parents. Their growth as individuals was given impetus by their adolescent years, and their search for a mate was also influenced by the experiences of those years.

Some parents thwart their child's movement toward emancipation and autonomy through their own doubts and insecurities. How they view themselves will affect how they relate to their children and especially how effective they will be in moving their children toward autonomy.

Modern-day stresses. So great are the day-to-day demands on parents that there is little time for them to contemplate their long-term goals and expectations. In addition, the dangers that parents must confront and overcome in guiding their children are so enormous that it seems eternal vigilance is required. These demands take away from parents' time to spend with their children, with each other, and by themselves.

Finding time for one's spouse, one's child, or oneself requires ingenuity at times. Unless the desire to find time exists, it won't happen. A structure is required to find time and a place to spend it. When desire is minimal and structure is excessive, the time will have an aura of artificiality and coercion.

Perhaps more important is a definition of what constitutes "quality time." Finding time is a challenge, but once such time is found, what is the quality to be? I've known mothers who held down a full-time job outside the home, took care of the home, and single-handedly raised their children to be healthy, happy, and well-adjusted. Time? Not much. Quality? High. Even a brief moment can be quality time. The following suggestions can help enhance the quality of time spent with children:

◆ Know how to listen in order to understand.
◆ Allow a child to talk about his or her feelings.
◆ Validate the child's feelings as legitimate.
◆ Express concern for the child and the problem.
◆ Inquire how one might help.

The amount of time is less important than the quality. Most parents have their own devices for making their available time count. The foregoing suggestions have more to do with parental attitude than with activities, and most parents know when time has been well spent.

A caveat: Find time for yourself. Tired, worn-out, unrefreshed parents will have difficulty in giving even one more ounce of energy or interest. Do your children a favor; give yourself time for refreshment.

Conclusion

Although adolescents bring their own strengths and weaknesses to their struggle toward adulthood, much of their ability to grow out of childhood is influenced by the psychological health of those who created, nourished, and nurtured them. Just as it is important for parents to understand what is happening to children, it is also important for parents to understand what is happening to themselves. Parents must do more than react to their children's needs. They must also take care of their own needs.

All of this is taking place within the context of the family. All family members are in the process of becoming whomever they are to be. Each member influences the developmental process of the other members and is influenced in return.

If the family is truly a psychological support system, it is within this context that we expect humans to prosper. It is in the environment of the family that we seek help during adversity. And it is here that children heal and grow. A healthy environment for children must promote growth toward individuality and connected autonomy. If that environment stifles growth, individuality, and connected autonomy for the parents, it will do the same to the children. It cannot be a wonderful place for children and yet a bad place for adults. To be a healthy place, all within must be allowed to grow and even to be helped in that growth.

Chapter 2

Adolescents and Their Parents

Although adolescents bring their own strengths and weaknesses to their struggle toward adulthood, much of their ability to grow out of childhood is influenced by the psychological health of those who created, nourished, and nurtured them.

In this chapter, I discuss adolescents' relationship with their parents from two sides: first, the changes in that relationship as the adolescent progresses toward adulthood, and second, guidelines for effective parenting that will help parents through all stages of their adolescents' development.

A Changing View of All-Powerful Parents

At the very beginning of life, children's existence depends upon the constant attention of dedicated caregivers who are not only willing but also powerful protectors. Without the ministrations of competent and willing caregivers, the newborn human infant would die. Based on the quality of care received, infants begin to form their first, highly significant impressions of the environment and the people who occupy it. These early impressions are made upon a yet unformed personality structure and will be embedded deeply in a child's unconscious mind. Later, the impressions are received into the conscious mind and will continually be reviewed and modified as a child grows; however, impressions on the unconscious for the most part remain hidden from continuing review.

As children progress into the preschool and school-age years, they project onto their parents qualities that, as helpless beings, they need to believe are available for their defense. In the course of psychological development, children's minds obtain the capacity for projection, projecting onto their parents an omnipotence and omniscience far beyond human capacity or even potential. Listen to the words of little children: "My father is the strongest man in the world." "My dad can beat your dad." "My mother is the most wonderful mother in the world. She loves me, she takes care of me," and so on. These beliefs are at the service of the developing ego and allow the vulnerable child to go merrily on his or her way, comfortable in the knowledge that he or she is safe from all harm.

Fighting the Myths in Adolescence

Once children approach adolescence, they begin to understand that they have acquired some power and knowledge. For example, a young male recognizes that now he is as tall as—if not taller than—his father. The adolescent female begins to measure herself against her mother, perhaps in physical measurements or in abilities: "Daddy says that my angel food cake is his favorite dessert." Adolescents certainly feel that they are smarter than their parents. But deep in the unconscious mind lurks the image of powerful parents and the image of a "poor, helpless me." Herein lies one of the more difficult conflicts adolescents and their parents must cope with as they progress through their respective life stages. If adolescents are to become fully autonomous and emancipated, they must begin to dismantle the belief that parents are all-powerful in order to free themselves of the belief that they are powerless. Adolescents must move toward parity in their view of themselves and their parents.

How does the adolescent accomplish this? Simple. Cut the ol' man down to size! Instead of now bragging, "My dad is the strongest man in the world!" the adolescent more than likely is saying, "My ol' man is a jerk. His views are pre–Civil War" or "My dad's unfair" or "My dad's . . . (you fill in the blanks)!" What is happening here is what I refer to as *demythologizing.* Adolescents now take back that which was given so long ago. They must now reclaim the power and knowledge for themselves in order to rid themselves of an image of helplessness.

As adolescents redefine their image of their parents, they fortunately also come to a discovery of their parents' humanness and a more sympathetic understanding of their parents' frailties. (Mark Twain commented on the enormous growth his father had undergone between Twain's sixteenth and twenty-second birthdays!) The time comes when parent and child complete their redefinition of each other. This involves neither triumph nor defeat, but a coming to terms.

Progress and the Associated Fears

Even though adolescents benefit from surrendering their long-held unconscious concepts of parents, it is nonetheless frightening for them to do so. As they relinquish the image of their parents as all-powerful and all-protecting, they must also give up the comfort of believing that they will always be safe from harm. This trade-off fills adolescents with ambivalent feelings that sometimes are played out in actions. Thus, just as an adolescent is making great strides toward maturity and increased responsibility, he or she might do something that prompts his or her parents into once again increasing their control over him or her, thereby reinstituting their protectiveness. Paradoxically, the adolescent then complains about that which he or she has invited. No wonder parents sometimes feel overwhelmed.

Consequences of Not Relinquishing an All-Powerful Image

Sometimes, an adolescent is unable to accept the redefinition of his or her parents as no longer being all-powerful and all-knowing. When parents unwittingly play into the all-powerful image, they are liable to foster their child's feelings of inadequacy and helplessness. Many adolescents experience guilt and anxiety about the disparaging of parents even in thought. Many of the control struggles between adolescent and parent find their origins here as the adolescent discovers covert ways of proving "you can't make me, so there!" Failing grades at school can be a consequence of an all-powerful parent's refusal to relinquish responsibility for the child's school performance. When this occurs, the child learns and perfects a host of behaviors designed to thwart powerful parents and console himself or herself that he or she is not powerless. The child will then likely become an adult who is fearful, angry, and secretly resentful. If this occurs, he or she is liable to have problems with authority figures and, for the most part, will maintain a poor self-image. Moreover, he or she will invite an ongoing parental concern because of what the parents perceive as the adult offspring's need to be protected. The young man or woman who maintains this helpless view of himself or herself will experience difficulty in meeting the demands that come with the establishment of a family and the requirement for becoming a provider of security in lieu of being a consumer of security.

A Long Process

It is important to understand the implications of adolescents' task of reformulating a view of their parents that is more consistent with an adult-to-adult relationship as they move toward autonomy. It is a task they must accomplish, but it is also one about which they have mixed feelings. They love their parents and sometimes feel guilty about their thoughts and behavior. But don't expect them to say so.

The process of demythologizing parents leads to a healthier and more realistic relationship, but not without anguish. The process lasts for several years but is not a constant source of trouble. It is not necessarily the initial endeavor of adolescence, but it is an important part of the process of adolescence.

I must emphasize that the process has far-reaching effects not only on the adolescent but also on those who love him or her. Even though turmoil need not accompany adolescence, the demythologizing process is of such importance that there is a potential for serious stress within the family. Much will depend upon how well the family is functioning at the time.

Effect of Demythologizing on Parents

The First Harbinger of Change

The adolescent's process of emancipation becomes a threat to the integrity of the family. Families have a life cycle: they are born, have an infancy, mature, grow old, and die. When the first adolescent begins to move away from his or her childhood, it is the first harbinger of the symbolic death of the family. Implicit in this first adolescent's successful move toward autonomy and independence lies the hidden message of the parents' fate: eventually the adolescent will no longer need his or her parents.

Parents of adolescent children are at a point in their lives when they are beginning to come to terms with their dreams, hopes, and ambitions. They may be approaching the height of their careers; now comes the time of great productivity, but limitations also begin to manifest themselves, options begin to narrow, and dreams of sudden fame and fortune are tempered by reality.

Derdeyn and Waters (1977) have written about how difficult it is for a father and son to develop a truly empathic understanding of each other. As a father observes his adolescent son, fresh in all of his glorious options, the father is reminded of the closing of his own options. The son, encumbered by his lack of experience, is hard pressed to understand the father's viewpoint, and the father, similarly blinded by his lack of inexperience, struggles to understand his son's viewpoint. For example, imagine the feelings of a 40-year-old father who, having had a bad day at the office the previous day and a restless sleep that night, comes downstairs to breakfast only to discover that he is a "jerk" in the eyes of his son. Although the father may intellectually understand his son's psychological struggles, it may not eliminate the tension that develops between him and his son after such an exchange.

Mid-life has challenges for fathers as well as mothers. Indeed, it has its challenges for nonfathers and nonmothers, widows, widowers, those who are divorced, and those who never married. Because I write about parents, I tend to pose these challenges in the context of parenthood, but they are confronted by all, parent or nonparent. Mid-life is a time to seek or maintain balance in one's life. It is a time to further reflect on the process of our sense of who and what we are as well as who and what we are becoming. For those who are parents, the bubble and squeak of the adolescent is such a ferment that it can absorb all of the energy of those in proximity.

A mother with an adolescent girl not only may face challenges in her work but also must confront the fundamental changes soon to take place in her physical and personal life. Although perhaps not yet menopausal, she has begun to see the approaching end of her reproductivity. Even though she might welcome the end of child-bearing, the event is one of considerable impact. Then, while all of this is in ferment, right under her nose blossoms her newly adolescent daughter, fresh in the beginning of her womanhood. It is an event that a mother celebrates but not without feeling some pain as she views the contrast between beginning and ending. A woman's ability to endure the loss of her reproductivity is intimately related to how she feels about herself as a woman and as an individual. In addition, as maternal demands lessen, she may find more energy to devote to herself, her needs, and to the other significant relationships in her life.

Parents' Reaction to Their Adolescent's New Independence

Although adolescents must begin to see their parents as less powerful, they do not want them to become powerless. Parents usually manage the transition with adequate grace. There are two potential dangers inherent in this process: too much done and too little done.

Some parents respond to their adolescent's "flexing muscles" of independence by clamping down or shortening the leash with which their child is tethered. Afraid that the child is going to get completely out of hand, a parent can send a negative message to the struggling child that he or she is not capable of becoming more responsible and thereby set up a self-fulfilling prophecy.

Equally unproductive is too little response. Parents, overwhelmed by the process, may throw up their hands in despair and give up. The parent who feels uncared for or not valued by his or her spouse is more likely to become enmeshed in a need-fulfilling relationship with his or her adolescent. Needing to feel valued, that parent might fail to apply limits rather than risk disapproval as a parent by the adolescent. The depressed parent—for whatever reason—is inclined to withdraw from conflicts that require much psychological energy.

Parents' Adjustment to Their Diminishing Role

As adolescents begin to reevaluate their unconscious concepts of parents, parents must, in turn, understand what is at stake. If being a parent represents the totality of a parent's life, then the loss of parenthood is going to be perceived as the end of life. The vast majority of the parents who have brought their troubled adolescents to me over the years had invested an overwhelming amount of their psychic and physical energy into their identities as parents and scarcely any as spouses. As their adolescents began redefining their unconscious concepts of their parents and began seeking emancipation, a very frightening message began to formulate in the minds of their parents. The movement toward adulthood meant the end of childhood, the end of childhood spelled the end of parenthood, and the end of parenthood spelled the end of everything.

Because of their anxiety about their changing role, parents become very concerned about their adolescent's future, but they also become concerned about their value and worth as a parent. Because they love their adolescent very much, they want his or her approval. Parents' need to be approved as parents becomes exaggerated if they feel unapproved of by their spouse or if they disapprove of themselves.

The adolescent's move toward emancipation should become a time of reevaluation and reflection for parents. As parenthood begins to end, parents begin to wonder, "After all these years together, besides our children, what do we have? What are we left with? When our adolescents leave, do we have nothing? Did we give it all to them?" Out of these questions comes an understanding that there are unspoken doubts that surface for parents.

For parents, the loss of their powerful role in the life of their adolescent is not a cause for rejoicing. Although at times trying, the role of parent is cherished. Even if not cherished, the role is a very serious responsibility for most. Surrendering the role of parent should not be equated with a dereliction of duty. It should not be a total surrender and certainly ought not be abrupt.

Parents Still Have a Role to Play

It is very important for parents to understand what lies behind some of their adolescent's actions. Because parents also have needs and may be attending to them, they might unwittingly fail to provide support for an adolescent's emancipatory efforts.

During the adolescent's efforts to reevaluate concepts of parents, both the adolescent and his or her parents experience loss. The adolescent loses all-powerful parents, and parents lose their "little boy" or "little girl." But each gains as well. The adolescent gains strength and a better self-image. He or she begins to seek a better image of himself or herself in relation to his or her parents and, in turn, in his or her relationship with other adults. The adolescent also seeks more responsibility and more control of his or her life. (One caveat: frequently, adolescents view their new station in life as a consequence of an increase in privileges rather than an increase in responsibility. Wise parents work toward the recognition that their adolescent wants more control but not total control.) Parents also gain. They gain a new relationship with a young adult and a new appreciation of their changing adolescent. These times bring great joy to parents. Making the psychological connection with their adolescent's emerging adultness is highly gratifying. "Somehow she (or he) is different; she (or he) just seems more grown up" is a happy observation shared by parents of grown adolescents.

Some Guidelines for Being an Effective Parent Through All Stages of Adolescence

Throughout the years, parents of my adolescent patients have beseeched me to give them the answer to ensuring success as parents.

They were seeking the list of "ten commandments of parenthood" that, if applied, would bring about parental salvation.

As I struggled to contemplate a list of do's and don'ts, I drew upon my experience with parents who had for the most part either not succeeded or succeeded in only a limited fashion in raising their children. I eventually concluded that there were many ways parents could disserve their children, but there was one almost universal failing among these dysfunctional families: the parents did not take care of each other!

Thus, the following points are offered as guidelines to parents struggling to understand their children and to help them grow to their potential. Many of these points are discussed in more detail elsewhere in this book.

✦ *Communication.* Feelings as well as facts should be clearly communicated. All family members should be allowed to express their opinions and ideas, as long as they accept responsibility for both their thoughts and their feelings. There should be an understanding that all members speak only for themselves and that they should not presume to speak for others. All communications should be responded to with respect for the individual expressing them.

✦ *Parental leadership.* Parents should provide clear, well-defined, *joint* leadership. In certain areas of family life the mother might be the agreed-upon leader, whereas in others the father might lead. The roles should be clear, consistent, and mutually agreed upon.

✦ *Discipline.* Parental authority, but not authoritarian behavior, should be clearly in operation. Children should have a clear understanding that the parents are in charge.

✦ *Self-responsibility.* Each family member should accept responsibility for his or her own behavior.

✦ *Respect for others.* Parents have the opportunity to model for their children conduct that shows respect for all others, especially for each other. In essence they are communicating to their children to "watch us and we will show you how human beings live together in an intimate relationship through caring and respect." If a father degrades his childrens' mother, what will they learn about women? If a mother ridicules her childrens' father, what will they learn about men? If parents fail to respect each other, what do children learn about self-respect?

✦ *Loving each other.* Each person wants to be loved and to matter to someone! Children who feel uncared for by parents seek acceptance elsewhere, and if they fail to find it, they become angry. The anger is then turned against the self and evolves into despair and despondency. These children begin to believe themselves unworthy of love if even their parents can't love them.

Maintaining the Boundary Between Being a Parent and a Friend

Some parents come to overvalue the role of friend and undervalue the role of parent. Wanting to maintain the approval of their children, parents may attempt to become their child's "best friend," which in reality is an uncritical good friend. Children can have many friends but only one mother and one father (except, of course, in the case of stepparents). Children must not be deprived of their parents because they have become simply another of their friends. Besides, what adolescent wants a best friend who is age 40?

The single parent is as likely as married parents, if not more likely, to become overwhelmed with the need to be a best friend, especially if he or she has unresolved feelings of guilt over the loss of the other parent.

Communicating Your Love to Your Child

All children want to be loved. Those who feel uncared for by parents seek love elsewhere; when they do not find it, they become angry, an anger that then evolves into despair and despondency. These children believe that they are unworthy of love because even their parents can't love them.

But sometimes, we're good parents in all ways except one: we cannot adequately communicate our love. We men seem to have more difficulty with this than is good for us. Some fathers are good husbands in all ways except expression of love. Fortunate are those husbands who, although inarticulate, are blessed with wives who know how to discern their love expressed in nonverbal ways. Many adolescents have complained to me that their fathers didn't love them. Their mothers assured me that it was not true. "He loves them very much but has trouble showing it," one mother declared. And almost invariably, he had trouble showing it to his wife, as well as his adolescent.

"But surely our child knows we love her!" is the fervent hope of parents. All parents. Even those who don't know how to show it. Do you and I "know" that we are loved? By our children? By our spouse? I believe that a wife wants to be valued not only as a mother but also as an individual, as a woman, and as a wife; similarly, a husband wants to be valued not only as a father but also as an individual, as a man, and as a husband. If a husband is too busy to show his wife that he cares about her, or if a wife is too busy to show that she cares about her husband, then their child is the real loser.

All parents love their child. But blessed are those who can and do express that love in both word and deed. Some might question the premise that *all* parents love their child; they might ask, "How can a parent do this or that if he or she truly loves his or her child?" My position is that all parents love their child, but I've never claimed that all parents are good parents.

I've seen parents who looked as if they didn't love, sounded as if they didn't love, or acted as if they didn't love their child. I've seen psychiatrically ill parents do horrible things to their children—abuse them, neglect them, destroy them. These are people who are sick. I've never known a psychologically mature, psychiatrically intact, well-adjusted, stable, and healthy child abuser!

Conclusion

Parents of today's adolescents have a responsibility to them. But indeed, we are the agents of transmittal for the values of society not only to our children but also to our children's children and future generations. In a risk-filled world, parents send their children forth with not much more than the distillate of their limited, hard-won wisdom and their prayers. They pray their children will be able to set their own limits on risk-taking behavior. By the time the children reach this point in their life, parents have given it their best shot. For most parents, children are eventually surrendered—grudgingly, perhaps, but finally.

Chapter 3

Communicating With Adolescents

John's parents sat on the sofa across from where he and I sat. They sat in silence as John talked incessantly to me. I would interject a question here and there for clarification. The parents sat in silence, with jaws hanging, and watched the interplay between their 15-year-old son and myself, a complete stranger. After 30 minutes, I stopped John, turned to his parents, and said, "I would like to hear your view of the problem." His father's first remark was, "I can't believe it! We had to practically drag him to your office. He told us we could make him come, but we couldn't make him talk. And here he sits gabbing away. I'm amazed at what you got out of him." In point of fact, I had "gotten" nothing out of him. He gave me an earful when I asked him to tell me his view of the problem. "All we can get out of him, Doctor, is 'I don't know' or else absolute silence," his mother added. "Whenever I try to talk to him, it ends up in a battle. He goes to his room, slams the door, and turns his music as loud as it will go. There is no communication between us. That is one of the reasons we brought him to see you. He won't communicate. And here he sits and talks and talks. Why?"

There were several reasons John talked with me. But perhaps the most important reason was that I was not his mother or father. Another reason was that I had trained myself to listen.

The Nature of Communication

There are two parts to all communication: content and process. *Content* embraces the words that are spoken and the ideas or feelings that are expressed; that is, what is being said. The *process* is what is not being said and is mostly transmitted nonverbally. The untrained observer will perhaps understand the content but will completely overlook the process. Understanding the process is somewhat speculative but also quite revealing, especially with regard to the relationship between the communicants. The process is a hidden message; one understands this message by doing what is somewhat akin to "reading between the lines." One of my predecessors referred to this as "listening with a third ear." What he was trying to convey is that people sometimes disguise their ideas and feelings and thus speak to one another in ways that are not always understood.

Take the following as an example. Mrs. A. is powdering her nose in the lady's room during an elegant affair. Mrs. B., standing beside her, asks: "Are those pearls real?" If we only listen to Mrs. A.'s words, we find out whether the pearls are real or not. On the other hand, if we listen to the words and watch the process, we'll not only discover the authenticity of the pearls, but we'll also learn how Mrs. A. feels about Mrs. B.'s asking this question. With shoulders back, head erect, and chin raised, Mrs. A. replies, "They certainly *are* real!" Thereby she validates the authenticity of the pearls and suggests that Mrs. B.'s question is an impertinence!

Knowing How to Listen

Listening With the Third Ear

Part of effective communication is the capacity to not just hear but to "listen." Over the years I gradually lost some of my physical ability to hear. I found myself having to focus my attention on the process of listening. I learned that I could not let my attention stray, even momentarily. I not only listened intently but also *conveyed the impression of* listening intently. Unintentionally, I drew benefits from my disability. An adolescent patient used to do a great imitation of me; his caricature drew heavily upon a face of intense scrutiny, head thrust forward, and hand cupped around the left ear. It really was funny. But the point is that I learned how to listen with more than just my ears.

I began to listen with my eyes as well. I learned that my adolescent patients would talk to me with their hands, their feet, their posture, their breathing, and their bodies. I learned that if I was going to understand them, I had to do more than merely listen. I had to watch closely. Sometimes a child would "tell" me how he felt by saying nothing. Sometimes I could glean information about how one patient felt by watching his or her reaction to what another said.

Listening in Order to Understand

Often people believe that all they need to do is talk with one another and everything will be alright. I've seen hundreds of adolescents and their families who "communicated"; that is, they talked and talked, but they still suffered in a variety of ways. Their problems seldom were caused by a lack of communication; they were almost always caused by a lack of understanding. They didn't really understand one another because they never heard one another. Oh, they listened, but they never listened the right way. Neither did I when I first began trying to understand adolescents. I listened. I heard everything they said. I could recite it back. And yet, although I was listening intently, I wasn't listening for the right purpose. It seemed that the harder I tried to hear everything, the less I heard.

In trying to hear everything, I interrupted too much and asked too many questions that began with a "why." In trying too hard, I conveyed my own anxiety and thus stimulated theirs. Once I recognized that it wasn't necessary to get every bit of information at that moment, I relaxed and so did they. Once I stopped "probing," they revealed more. Once I mastered the belief that no patients want to feel that they must "tell all" and be stripped of all of their hidden thoughts, I was able to believe and to convey the idea of "tell me about that *if you can*." Knowing that they didn't *have* to tell me, they were then *able* to tell me. Responding to their efforts to talk about something frightening or shameful, I needed to rein in my parental anxiety and avoid responding with "You did WHAT?" or "Now, WHY in the world would you do such a thing?"

We all respond positively to the good listener who seems genuinely interested in our ideas or opinions and who treats those expressions with respect rather than with ridicule or abrupt refutation. Some of the things an adolescent says might need refutation at some point, but not while one is trying to get the adolescent to overcome his or her fear of sharing information. My responses to the adolescent who was trying to talk were such that let him or her know that I was interested in hearing more. "I see." "Umm." "Umm Hmm." "Oh?" "That's interesting!" "How did you feel when that happened?" "Gosh, that must have been scary!" The foregoing comments conveyed three things to my young patients:

1. I am listening.
2. I am interested in learning how the world appears through your eyes.
3. Tell me more if you can.

I believe that parents invest considerable energy in trying to understand their children, especially the adolescent. But a great deal of that energy misses the mark. Adolescents often believe their parents don't understand them because their parents do not listen to what they say. The problem is that parents frequently are planning their rebuttal to what is being said and can hardly wait to tell their adolescent children why they don't know what they are talking about. Too frequently parents are intent on "setting them straight" rather than simply trying to understand what they are attempting to say. They might need to be set straight, but if that's all a parent is interested in doing, it will be quite apparent, and that parent will be perceived as not listening.

Listening to Adolescents

Some of the things adolescents tell me are difficult to listen to, some are naive, some are silly, some are boring, and some scare me.

I also find that so many of the adolescent's thoughts, ideas, and verbal productions could use corrections. Some could do with outright refutation. And yet, I must do all I can to help them tell me about the terrifying thoughts that enter their minds. If I am to have a chance of hearing what is in their minds, I must listen with only one objective: simple and unadorned understanding. I am concerned with the process of listening and trying to understand how the one I am listening to came to believe such an idea rather than with the validity of the idea.

Confirming Your Understanding of Adolescent Communication

Because adolescents are easily misunderstood, I go about the process of listening very carefully. I remind myself that all I'm supposed to do right now is to make sure that I understand what they are saying. So I try to keep my mouth shut while they talk to me. After each sentence, I nod my head or raise my eyebrows or utter some noncommittal sound, none of which suggests that I agree or disagree; these responses simply suggest that I'm listening. After four or five sentences, I'll interrupt and say, "Let me see if I understand what you are trying to say. From what I hear you saying, I get the impression that you believe. . . ." My questions to them begin with, "Let me see if I understand." I then restate in my own words what I think has been said. They are then in a position to say, "No, that is not what I'm trying to tell you. What I'm trying to say is . . ." or else they agree that I have heard correctly what has been said. So far, I haven't agreed or disagreed. All I've done is suggest that what they are saying is important enough for me to listen to carefully. What is of primary importance is whether I respect them enough to listen carefully. These adolescents are trying to tell me what it is like to be them.

Adolescents' Nonverbal Communication

Communicating with adolescents is not always easy—not for adults and not for adolescents. Sometimes it seemed to me that no matter what I said, nothing worked. So I would be quiet. And then, some would talk. Some answered my questions only with a shrug of the shoulders. I eventually learned that a shrug meant one of the following:

◆ I do not have the information you are seeking.
◆ I have the information, but it's none of your business.
◆ I am afraid to answer.

Sometimes, at what seemed a critical juncture of the session, a young adolescent patient would yawn. I would be tempted to interpret this as boredom and thus feel offended. Sometimes it meant that he or she was bored. But sometimes it meant that last night this child spent the night tossing and turning from horrible dreams. Some had wept all night. Some were very depressed.

Another way the adolescent might speak nonverbally is by not speaking at all. The deadly silence might speak eloquently of anger, but it might also be the equivalent of "I have great trouble talking, especially to adults and authority figures."

Hidden Meanings

Adolescents are not the world's greatest communicators, and some of the things they say are almost unintelligible, even without their slang. Large portions of my humility have come as a consequence of realizing that just when I begin to think that I understand them, they remind me that I don't.

What the adolescent means is sometimes hidden from view and must be sought, because the real meaning can be quite revealing. Let me cite an exchange that took place between me and one of my patients on the adolescent ward one morning:

Dan, a 14-year-old boy who had been physically and emotionally abused in life, was brought to the hospital after a suicide attempt. He seemed to be responding positively to the security of his new environment. He let the nurses know that he liked feeling safe. However, he was distant with me, and, despite my efforts to get something going with him, he remained apart.

As I entered the ward one day, I spoke to several adolescents near the entrance. I turned to see Dan glaring at me. "You don't like me!" he declared in a most unfriendly manner. My first impulse was to feel offended. My second impulse was to defend myself against this unfair accusation, saying something like, "What do you mean saying something like that to me after all the hard work I've done to help you? Who do you think has been trying to make things better for you? Is that the thanks I get?" and so on. Instead, I decided to seek the hidden meaning in his words. I was confused and said to him, "I don't understand." His reply was, "Yes you do, you don't like me!" I asked: "I don't? You believe that I don't like you?" "That's right," he snapped. "Gosh, Dan, what is it that I'm doing that would cause you to feel that way?" I asked. "You spoke to everybody else and didn't speak to me!" he informed me. "Oh, I see! I guess I'd feel the same way if I thought someone didn't want to speak to me. How does it make you feel thinking that your own doctor doesn't like you?" I inquired. "It scares me. It makes me think that you might send me away," was his almost whispered response. "I'm not going to send you anywhere, Dan, not until you and I both think it's time to go," I assured him. I touched his shoulder and said no more.

Initially, I had been tempted to refute Dan's statement. Instead, I chose to find out what had prompted his statement. My obvious struggle to understand what was going on in this unhappy young man made a statement to him far more eloquent than a defensive denial of his charge. I didn't have to tell him I cared about him. He concluded that on his own.

I was fortunate that Dan was willing to give me bad news. Too frequently, children will misinterpret parental actions and feel hurt, but out of "respect" they keep it to themselves. If they tell us about it, we have a chance to put it right. Whether they are willing to bring unpleasant news to us depends upon how we ordinarily react to bad news.

Communicating: An Anxiety-Producing Experience for Many Adolescents

Early on in my practice, I learned that talking can be an anxiety-provoking experience for adolescents. I can think of one patient in particular who found communicating difficult. All manner of confusing things were welling up inside this boy. He heard hallucinatory voices urging him to kill himself. Thinking about these things was frightening to him, and he felt that talking about them would surely make them come true. I needed to know what was going on inside his head if I was going to help him. I was so eager to help him that I tried to drag it out of him. Well, I learned that trying to drag answers out of him produced the opposite effect: silence. It is always easier to talk if you don't have to. Once this concept became clear to me, I realized that I could help this adolescent manage his anxiety by first managing my own. As I relaxed, so did he.

Knowing how to listen is important, but encouraging an adolescent to talk comes before listening. I must convey an interest in hearing what's on his or her mind without scaring him or her half to death. I must remember that my listening will help the adolescent feel better, but I must be patient. He or she might not want to talk when I am ready to listen. My saying something like, "That's alright. Talk about it when you can. I'll be here to listen," can be helpful.

When an adolescent—or adult—is trying to talk about something extremely difficult, a sympathetic comment can help. Sometimes adolescents, on the verge of tears, will struggle to hold back their words for fear they will overflow. It is encouraging to say something like, "Sometimes it is difficult to talk about these things, and if you can't talk, I'll try to understand. But sometimes it helps. It can help you feel better, and it can help me understand." I've been surprised at how well the adolescent responds when I am willing to keep my mouth shut and my eyes and ears open.

When adolescents are in the midst of some sort of disagreement with one or both parents, their anxiety increases, and their verbal skill decreases. If the questions put to them demand answers that will demean them in their own image of themselves, they will frequently shut down and refuse to talk, not necessarily because they are guilty, but because anxiety makes talking impossible.

One thing to remember is that help isn't always helpful. Sometimes parents themselves are trying to help, particularly if they are worried to death about what is happening to their child. Sometimes the recipients of "help" don't call it help.

Adolescents' Difficulty in Talking With Adults

In many ways, communication with adolescents is no different from communication with adults. What makes communication with adolescents difficult is that their verbal skills are not yet fully developed and that they experience anxiety when talking with adults.

One of my adolescent patients complained to me about his relationship with his parents. "I can't talk to my parents," he grouched. I replied, "Come on, Peter, I've heard that complaint from adolescent after adolescent. You make it sound as if your parents won't let you talk with them. I've talked with your parents, and frankly, I find them open and ready to listen." He shook his head and said, "Sure, *you* can, but *I* can't!" I then realized that what this patient was talking about was not a defect he found in them but one which he found in himself. Perhaps that was what all those other adolescents meant. In his sentence "I can't talk to my parents" the explanation lay in the first three words: "I can't talk."

The process of adolescence itself makes communication with adults difficult. All of adolescents' struggle to leave their childhood and move to adulthood greatly colors their communication. They are extremely sensitive to any suggestion that they are still children, particularly in the eyes of their parents. The main reason I can communicate with patients' parents is because I am not their little boy or little girl. There is no dependency struggle going on between me and them. I do not need to prove to them that I am no longer a child. I am not trying to free my mind of idealized images of these parents. I am not struggling to come to terms with who I am.

Teaching Adolescents How to Disagree With Respect

One 15-year-old boy got into a heated discussion with his father and during the exchange raised his voice and shouted at his father. His father shouted back, "Don't you dare talk to me like that young man!" The boy fell silent, began to weep and said, "I'm sorry, but Dad, if I can't talk with you when I'm upset, who can I talk to?" His father suddenly realized that it was difficult to be upset and speak calmly. His son was not being disrespectful, only loud.

Communication with the adolescent might very well become loud at times, which I don't mind. But I will not tolerate obscenities or demeaning terms (e.g., fatty, skinny, jerk, dumb-dumb) from adolescents. And I will not use either in my communication with them. If adolescents use profanity in communication with me, I tell them that I'm offended and that I would appreciate it if they would not do that again. I have been impressed with how considerate the adolescent can be when treated with respect. I urge parents to avoid using profanity with adolescents and to simply not allow them to do so. Moreover, do not allow them to belittle or demean you.

There are ways to express feelings verbally without being offensive. I expect angry children to look angry and sound angry. I urge them to develop their vocabulary so as to be able to describe a broad range of anger from "irritated" to "upset" to "furious" to "livid with anger" to "enraged" and to use the most appropriate descriptor as they verbally rather than behaviorally express their feelings.

Encouraging Adolescents to Express Both Positive and Negative Feelings

In too many families, only nice feelings can be expressed. Adolescence can be a time of extreme stress and a time of terrible feelings. Too often, adolescents believe that they should keep those feelings inside. They actually believe that they shouldn't get angry and that if they do feel anger they should count to 10 and then the anger will disappear. It disappears, of course, only to be buried deep down inside of them where they no longer feel it. But deep inside, the anger lurks. Eventually, when someone else provokes that anger, the adolescent responds with an explosive outburst that is disproportionate to the offending action. This outburst is followed by remorse and embarrassment and then by a resolve to not get angry ever again.

Communication of ideas is important, but even dysfunctional families usually allow such. It's the communication of affects or feelings that is more frequently forbidden. Being able to talk with another human being about frightening feelings is critical to the maintenance of one's mental health. Being able to legitimize these feelings through the discovery of their existence in others is a fundamental premise in psychotherapy. Being able to express feelings in words rather than combat is a major step for the child trying to become an adolescent and the adolescent trying to become an adult.

Gaining Reassurance From Adolescents

As a psychiatrist who treats adolescents, I must struggle to earn what parents usually already have: their adolescent's trust! I do that when I treat that adolescent with respect. Then, as I gain his or her trust, I become a valued person to him or her, and my ideas and ideals, when, at the right time, I share them with him or her, will take on value.

Parents are already valued people to their adolescent, but often they don't realize that. For example, adolescents, for the most part, adopt their parents' basic values. But parents constantly doubt their effectiveness with their children. One reason is that children seldom reassure them with the validations parents so diligently seek. I've not known many adolescents who felt it necessary to periodically declare, "Gee, Mom and Dad, I want to assure you that you are doing a very good job. You're a fine mother, and you're a fine father." They can't say such things. Besides, what do they know about parenting? But a great part of parental frustration arises from the poor communication parents have with their adolescent. There are ways to make that better. Learning how to listen will help.

Guidelines for Communicating With Adolescents

Communicating with an adolescent is often a challenge. He or she is struggling with changes in his or her life, and parents are struggling to understand their changing child. The following are some guidelines to encouraging meaningful communication between parent and child:

1. *Talking will be easier if it is your adolescent's idea.* It's difficult to gleefully and enthusiastically "chat" against one's wishes.

When a conversation is a "command performance," expect some balking. Adolescents will be more willing to talk when it's their idea. Timing is important in that they might not be able to talk about something touchy at the moment you want them to. Let them know that you want to talk with them, but if they feel that they can't talk at that particular time, you will be available when they feel they can talk. Of course, follow up.

2. *Be yourself in conversations with your adolescent.* If you want to keep communication open with your adolescent, try to keep the setting informal and relaxed. But be what you are—an adult! Some adults foolishly believe that by being adolescent in dress, behavior, and conversation they will gain some sort of credibility with the younger generation. Not so. When adolescents observe adults (especially parents) posing as adolescents, they lose the adult model they so desperately need in their pursuit of adulthood. And worse, the adult appears phony! On the other hand, it's not helpful to be a pompous stuffed shirt. Be natural, but be yourself. Having reached adulthood, we should have left behind our adolescence.

3. *Be honest in presenting your view.* Call a spade a spade. Lies ought not to be called "fibs," and stealing ought not to be called "taking things." Parents ought not to tempt children to lie by asking, "Did you do this?" when the parent knows for a fact that the child did do it. An honest declaration such as, "I know that you did this. Don't do it again, or you'll be punished," is telling it like it is.

I recall an adolescent patient who was capable of making above-average grades in school and who described his two Cs and three Ds as "not too good." I agreed that they certainly were not "in excess of good." I suggested that a description of "disgraceful" would be more correct. He agreed.

4. *Ask questions that encourage answers.* If parents seek better communication with their adolescent, they should let their questions begin with "How do you feel about . . .?" or "In your opinion, what causes . . .?" Some questions are easier to answer than others. Some are very difficult to answer. "What makes you so stupid?" is the type of question that generates little in the way of enthusiastic response. One of my contemporaries

many years ago earned himself a whack from his father who had asked him this very same question. His father didn't think much of my friend's answer: "Heredity!" "Why are you so stubborn? so bad? so sassy?" and so on fall in the category of questions no one wishes to answer. Another question, "Why did you do that?" demands a justification for what one has done. It says, "Give me one good reason!" There may be no justification that will be acceptable to the questioner.

The "Why did you do that?" questions are more difficult to answer than ones that begin "How did you . . .?" For example, "How did you feel when you broke your word to your mom?" is more likely to get a response than "Why did you break your word to your mom?" "How do you think she felt about that?" puts the focus where it should be, in that it helps the respondent answer rather than simply putting him or her on the defensive.

Often, questions are hidden behind other questions. A father and his son were discussing the legality of marijuana use. The words they used dealt mostly with the drug, but what was not being asked was, "Who is in charge here?" A mother and her 16-year-old daughter were having a heated discussion about the reputation of the daughter's boyfriend. What was not being asked from the daughter's side was, "Who will run my life?" From the mother's side, it was "It's my duty to keep you from harm."

5. *Let your adolescent talk.* If you want to get information from your adolescent, let him or her talk. If you want to give information, you do all the talking. This is a process that is difficult to master. Sometimes when parents are upset with their adolescent, it is hard not to run on and on with demands of "Why did you?" or "Why didn't you?" Knowing how to listen makes it easier for your child to talk with you. It's not easy for adolescents to talk with adults, and, sometimes, it is even more difficult for them to talk with parents. But adolescents will never talk if the parents go on and on. If you must interrupt, do so only to clarify. Questions such as, "Let me see if I understand what you're trying to say," followed by "If I understand correctly, you're trying to tell me that I don't . . .," not only are

permissible but also convey the impression that you are trying to understand what your child is trying to say. Otherwise let him or her finish and then ask, "Is that all? Is there anything else you need to tell me?"

6. *Try to avoid lectures.* This especially applies to those lectures that your adolescent has already listened to. Tell them what you think and feel. "It makes me angry when you . . ." or "I'd appreciate it if you would not do that again" or "It hurts my feelings when you ignore me." Skip the "Don't you realize. . . ." approach. Long dissertations on "Why, when I was your age, I. . . ." or lectures on "how tough it was back then" will terminate adult-adolescent communication quicker than anything else. Such remarks are heard by the adolescent as, "Let me tell you how weak you are. Let me tell you how my generation invented virtue, how my generation preferred hardships to comfort. We volunteered for deprivation so as to build character," and so on.

7. *When disciplining, talk about assets as well as liabilities.* If you are going to point out unacceptable behavior, do it in the context of contrasting the unacceptable aspects of your adolescent's behavior with the more admirable qualities he or she usually presents. Adolescent hearing is improved if our comments can begin with good news. "You know, Jack, you're usually so thoughtful of others, I'm surprised at the way you treated your sister. I'm disappointed. That's not like you," is more easily integrated into his concept of himself than, "There you go; you never think of anyone but yourself. Shame on you for treating your sister that way!" Adolescents have blemishes. But they also have their attractive qualities and feel proud when they hear parents recognize them.

8. *Recognize the difference between words and behavior.* Some of the things adolescents tell me scare the daylights out of me. Some of the ideas they express are radical and extreme; for the most part, they are idealistic. Adolescents' idealism is at least partly due to the fact that they don't have many years of experience in the school of hard knocks. Their political ideas are bound to generate heat. They will be pleasantly surprised if you refuse to belittle their opinions. They really don't expect you to agree

with them and secretly hope you won't. But they want to use their newly found skills of abstract thinking. Don't be alarmed if their comments sound antiestablishment, radically liberal, or even nihilistic. One of the reasons they express such ideas is to get a "rise" out of adults. I worry more about adolescent behavior than I do about adolescent opinions. Opinions expressed are not the same as behavior acted out. When the adolescent says, "I think they should legalize marijuana," it does not necessarily mean "I'm going to start smoking pot!"

9. *Respect your adolescent's confidence.* Discussing the matter with your mate is proper. Discussing the adolescent's problem with siblings is not. Respecting what adolescents tell you means treating the information with sympathy and dignity and refusing to use the information to ridicule or degrade. But have an understanding with your mate—and make clear to your children—that neither of you will collude with them to keep the information secret from your spouse. To do so is bad for your marriage and bad for their impression of your relationship with your spouse. One of the problematic aspects of dysfunctional families is their tendency toward collusions and secrecy.

   If the information is serious enough that it be shared with the other parent, let your child be the one to tell the other parent. Let your child know that you will go with him or her and help, but that he or she must do the telling. "If you are absolutely unable to tell your Dad, then I will be compelled to tell him, but you will have to be there when I do," states the issue clearly.

10. *You're probably doing better than you think.* Try not to be invasive. Give them some distance. It's not necessary that you know everything. Trying too hard can end the process of communication. None of us wants to feel stripped bare and robbed of all of our secrets.

Parents Need to Communicate With Each Other

Parents need to communicate with each other as they cope with their child's movement through adolescence, because this process also brings on changes for parents. For example, a parent's recognizing that his or her child is moving away from him or her toward independence and autonomy can bring not only happiness but also fear and sadness. A parent's ability to share those feelings with someone who loves him or her can augment the happiness and diminish the fear and sadness; a parent's relationship with his or her spouse or significant other can provide just the caring relationship needed for such sharing.

Conclusion

Communication between two people is influenced by the relationship between them. Enormous forces are at work in adolescents' lives, and these forces will color the relationships they have with the important people in their lives. If parents have some understanding of the psychological challenges their adolescent is trying to master, it will help clarify and improve the communication.

Parents' communication with their adolescents should lead to an understanding of each other. As adolescents begin to pull away from the protection of the family, they must take with them a set of values that is designed to help them live in harmony with their world. Those values should be real and should help adolescents impose upon themselves limits to their instinctual urges. The capacity for self-discipline must begin before adolescence. It becomes critical during adolescence. If clear boundaries and limits have been communicated to adolescents before their departure from the safety of the family, they will take with them an ability to impose those limits upon themselves as they embark into a world of risk.

Chapter 4

Setting Limits for Adolescents

~~~~~~

*S*o many misunderstandings between parents and adolescents revolve around the matter of control. Control becomes a central theme of adolescence and hides itself in many struggles that do not at first appear to involve control issues, as in the following example:

> Ellie, a 17-year-old girl, was brought to me by her parents because of her symptoms of depression, but also because of heated battles between her and her mother. "I don't care what she says, I'm not going to approve of her relationship with that boy James," her mother assured me. "He is trash; he has been kicked out of school, uses drugs, sells drugs, and is currently on probation for breaking and entering. On top of all of that, he is emotionally and physically abusive to Ellie. He is the reason Ellie and I fight so much!"
>
> Ellie's view of James was at odds with that of her mother. "The trouble is, Mother, you're a snob! His family is poor, and they don't live in the country club. His mother has problems and uses drugs. He has trouble learning in school. . . ."
>
> I was inclined to share the mother's concern about the boy who she feared might become her future son-in-law, but as I listened to these two people fight, I realized that they were not fighting the same battle. To the mother, the issue was that she must save Ellie from a horrible fate. To Ellie, the issue was not James, but rather her mother's control—"She is trying to run my

53

life!" For her mother, the issue was protecting Ellie, which was interpreted by Ellie as her mother's wanting to control her. In her struggle to shed the image of a helpless little girl, Ellie felt that she dare not give in to her mother's demands. In some ways, Ellie needed to hang on to James in order to prove to herself and her mother that she was no longer a little girl.

As soon as Ellie's mother understood the hidden agenda in their fighting, she was able to restructure her position. "I love you, Ellie, and sometimes I'm inclined to try to protect you, whereas you are really the only one who can do that. You know my feelings about James. I think he is a nice-looking fellow, but he has some serious problems that may yet destroy him. I'd rather you find someone with a better future." Thus, the control issue was defused. Ellie no longer needed to continue seeing James and subsequently discontinued the relationship. Although she resented her mother's attempt to control her, she was confused by the good feelings generated in her when her mother talked about protecting her.

Adolescence as a Period of Increased Responsibility

Adolescence is thought of as a period of responsibility adjustment. Adolescents must become more responsible for their behavior and parents less responsible for their adolescent's behavior. Control of adolescent behavior must shift away from parents and toward the adolescent—but not completely.

Increased Difficulty in Controlling Adolescents

By the time they reach adolescence, young people are big enough, skilled enough, and mobile enough that they are very difficult to control. With that mobility, they become mercilessly vulnerable to unlimited danger. Just thinking about this scares most parents. But how can parents protect them without controlling them? They can't! Only adolescents can protect themselves, but they might not! This is the most unpleasant experience of parenthood, this sense of helplessness that comes to the parents of adolescents. For the first time in their life, they are no longer able to control their offspring and consequently are no longer able to protect them.

And the wretched part of it all is that parents believe that somehow they are failing in the central mission of parenthood. Enormous servings of guilt seem a steady diet for parents at this stage of life. Somehow the self-nagging continues in their belief that they should be able to protect their adolescent and that they could do so if only they were clever enough.

Increased Risk and Increased Consequences for Adolescents

As adolescents become more capable of indulging in risk-taking behavior (see Chapter 8), they are more vulnerable to its consequences. Limit setting becomes a critical issue around the time of emancipation and freedom from direct parental supervision of behavior. Moreover, the focus of control *should* begin to shift toward adolescents because they are reaching a point in their lives when they are going to be held personally accountable for their actions— perhaps by school authorities, perhaps by the police, perhaps by the grim reaper. With more and more crimes being committed by young adolescents, society is losing its patience and its sentimentality toward youthful offenders. Still protective of the very young child, courts are beginning to view older adolescents as accountable for their behavior. It is not in the adolescent's best interest to continue believing that "Mommy and Daddy will be held accountable instead of me" or that "Mommy and Daddy will save me."

Reasons for Adolescents' Resisting Parental Control

Recently, while in the process of writing this book, I was approached by a gentleman whose face was familiar. He smiled, extended his hand, and said,

> I'm Jim B. and you treated my son 15 years ago. You helped him, but I think you helped me even more. You helped me learn that I was responsible for the behavior of just one person—me! I learned that there was only one person I could control—me! My son is getting along just fine and so am I. Thank you.

This father had felt the way most parents feel, that somehow or another he had to keep his son from all harm, but he had eventually come to realize that he could not control his son's behavior. When parents believe they must still control their adolescent, they embark on a course of actions that thrusts them into the role of controllers. They may not realize this; they simply love their children and want the best for them.

Unwittingly, when parents take on the role of controllers, they cast their adolescent in the role of controllees. Because of the underlying dynamics of adolescent behavior, it becomes, in the adolescent's mind, imperative that he or she resists. Failure to resist means a return to the time when he or she was a helpless child. Because adolescents love their parents and need them, they find themselves in a dilemma. Resisting parental control puts them in a battle with their parents; meekly acquiescing to parental control results in their losing face with themselves and feeling withdrawn, depressed, and helpless. Resisting can become a substitute for helplessness.

How to Set Limits

Any discussion of setting limits for the adolescent should be entered into carefully and with the recognition that sometimes it seems that nothing works. It is an area of parenthood that can be very frustrating.

Necessity of Setting Limits Early in Children's Lives

Young children's safety lies in the hands of those who care for them, and thus it is important that early on parents impose restrictions that are designed to keep their children safe from harm. Setting limits should have the child's safety and welfare in mind, as well as the safety and welfare of those who must share the environment. Rules for children should be simple and attainable, but even more important, they should be communicated in a clear, concise, and consistent manner.

The reasons for setting these limits early in the child's life are that the child is so vulnerable early in life and that this is a critical time in the child's measurement of his or her environment and those who inhabit that environment. At this time, a capacity for trust will develop in either a healthy or a flawed way. That capacity will play a significant role in the child's personality development and might come to color his or her adolescent and adult capacity for trust in others. And it serves the young child well in the formulation of his or her concepts of the parents' ability to protect. If a young child sees the parents as too weak to control him or her, he or she also sees the parents as being too weak to protect him or her.

Some Rules About Setting Rules

1. *The content, and not the number, of rules is most important.* Parents should coalesce their philosophies into a coherent set of the most important rules, rules that both parents can support. For example, central to parental responsibility is the preservation of one's child's life. Whatever behavior you permit or forbid, ask, "If I allow my child to do this, is there significant risk to her or his life?" If the answer is yes, then do whatever you can to forbid it. If the answer is no, then ask this follow-up question: "Is this an issue that is central to the building of my child's development of character?" For children to become fully functional as adults, they must develop the qualities that will help them get along with their family, friends, and co-workers (see list of desirable qualities enumerated below in the subsection, "How have we done so far in raising our child?"). Parents' ability to set and implement reasonable rules, administered lovingly and consistently, will add the critical component of respect for authority.
2. *Rules should have value.* Rules ought not to be capricious. Moreover, they should be genuine. Parents ought not to impose rules that they do not respect. Rules become valueless if you are not prepared to back them up.
3. *Rules should have a purpose.* Although all individuals must face the consequences of their behavior, adolescents have not yet had vast experiences from which they can draw a solid sense of

cause and effect. Rules should have a purpose, and the purpose should include the establishment of behavioral responses that will help adolescents adapt to their environment and their fellow human beings. Adolescents must discover that when they do X, Y will happen, and that if they don't like Y, then perhaps they shouldn't do X. With the assumption of adulthood, all begin to take on the responsibility of abiding by a wide variety of rules imposed by society as well as by self-imposed rules.

4. *Rules should be clearly stated.* Parents should clearly communicate their expectations to their children concerning the way they behave at home, work (school), and play. Rules should be simple to follow. Both parents should share both in the making of the rules and in their implementation. If a parent has mixed feelings about a rule, his or her ambivalence will be apparent to his or her child. There should be no ambiguity concerning parents' expectations.

5. *Rules should be limited in number.* Determine which areas are the most essential for limit setting. Successful governments avoid micromanagement and allow their citizens the privilege and responsibility of determining the majority of their actions. Parents have their hands full with enough responsibilities without having to make sure that they control all of their children's behavior.

Some children seem to want a highly structured environment, whereas others do better with fewer rules. Some parents are inclined toward a high degree of strictness, whereas others are more permissive. I have treated children from highly disciplined homes as well as those from highly permissive homes. When taken to excess, each environment can be maladaptive. An overly strict environment can produce nervous or inhibited children. An environment with no rules might produce children who feel unsafe and confused.

Look upon each rule imposed as work for the parents. The more rules, the more work. Some parents are so encumbered with multiple rules that they spend all of their time in the micromanagement of their child's life—time that must come from their other pursuits and from their relationship with each other. Moreover, multiple rules tend to contaminate the relationship with one's children by casting it as an ongoing adversarial struggle.

6. *Rules should help adolescents "not cross the line."* Parents must think carefully about the rules imposed on their young. When they draw the line for their child, they are suggesting that beyond that line is where danger lies. But they are also suggesting that safety lies within the borderline set by the parents. Knowing where danger lies helps us avoid it.

   For example, an invading army always crosses a minefield after a pathway has been staked out and clearly identified with markers. Each soldier knows that within these boundaries, everything is safe. If those soldiers suddenly see a group of other soldiers scampering about in what is supposed to be unsafe territory, they are going to have second thoughts about where safety lies.

7. *Children will test rules.* They do so to assure themselves that parents mean what they say. When a child tests the line, he or she should experience immediate consequences, whatever those might be. The child's act of testing the line might seem mischievous and calculating to his or her parents. "It's almost as if he wants me to punish him," one frustrated mother declared. "He pushes me and pushes me until I finally blow up at him. And then he behaves. It's almost as if he enjoys seeing me angry!" Not so, I say. What her son enjoyed was discovering where safety lies. If breaking the rule offers no danger, then keeping the rule offers no safety.

8. *Stick by your word.* In the days of the old West, people lived by a simple rule: "Don't reach for your gun unless you intend to shoot!" In the same vein, I am suggesting "Don't promise (or threaten) and not mean it!" Your rules should be predictable and consistent. Keeping your word and delivering on promises makes an enduring impression on children. It models for them the value of reliability. Promises ought not to be issued carelessly. If we say we will, we must!

   So much is changing for adolescents that they seek things that they can depend upon. They want the list of rules to be shortened, but they don't expect or want all to be removed. With only a few rules—important rules—to back up, parents have a great opportunity to present themselves as dependable and predictable. I recall an adolescent complaining to a friend "Aw, it won't do any good, she's already said, 'You're not going out on that sailboat in this kind of weather.' It wouldn't do any good to beg; she never changes her mind about things like that!" All of this was said with frustration but not without a degree of relief.

9. *When appropriate, change the rules.* Children grow, and as they do, their needs change. Their ability for self-governance increases with their maturing sense of personal responsibility. Parental recognition of that growing maturity should lead to a change in the rules. As soon as your adolescent is willing and able to relieve you of the onerous task of running his or her life, let him or her do so. With increased self-responsibility goes increased self-determination.

Guidelines are nothing more than that. They merely guide. The foregoing discussion amounts to mere suggestions and offers opportunities to review concepts that were already learned but perhaps that were shoved aside in the day-to-day struggle to be a good parent. Use them if they make sense to you.

How to Enforce Limits

Withdrawal of Parental Approval

Most children will surrender any gratification to maintain the approval of a loving parent. Sometimes, the most effective "punishment" is the calmly stated declaration, "Son, I am disappointed with what you did. I am angry about it, but mostly I am disappointed. It's not like you to be irresponsible. You've let me down, but more importantly, you've let yourself down. I'd like to see you straighten this matter out." These are my words—yours might be better—but they express genuine feelings. They are not belittling or demeaning. They express disapproval of behavior, while saying something positive about the child. If you have a good relationship with your child, these words will be very effective. If you don't have a good relationship, these words will catch your child off guard and will offer an opportunity to improve that relationship.

Some parents are comfortable and effective with such an approach, whereas others prefer loss of privileges. Clarity and consistency are critically important because they bring predictability into the child's life.

Rules for Enforcing Rules

When parents jointly have decided on the rules they wish to impose on their children, they must then confront the issue of how to enforce those rules. As mentioned above, the most important guideline is consistency—applying rules to all children equally and applying consequences to broken rules without deviation. The following three guidelines help to maintain this consistency:

1. *Be sure your rules are enforceable.* Predictions about what you are going to do if your child doesn't do such and such need to be thought out in advance as to the likelihood of your being willing and able to make your prediction come true.

   Fred Junior's father was a large man. He was quiet and easygoing and tended to avoid conflict. Mama was the opposite: she was petite, intense, conscientious, and energetic. At age 14, Fred Junior was 6'2" and weighed just under 200 pounds. One Saturday morning his mother became frustrated that her son was still in bed at 10:00 A.M. She was certain that such indolence would lead to a life of sloth and did her best to "nag" him out of bed or at least ruin his sleep! "If you don't get out of that bed this instant," she demanded, "I am going to pull you out!" Fred Junior stretched out his huge frame, put his hands behind his head, and said, "Pull!" Later, the mother fumed to me, "There was no way that I could pull him out of his bed, so I struck my colors and retreated." Although angry with Fred Junior, she was furious with Fred Senior for not being more upset about their son's lack of "get up and go."

   On the other hand, I have seen mothers look up into the eyes of a taller son and deliver a demand that was quickly met, not because of the son's respect for his mother's physical strength, but because of his respect for her moral strength, her love, and her predictability. These mothers' demands were never unreasonable; their rules were few, logical, and well supported by their mate. If rules were broken, there had always been sanctions imposed, even if only a verbal expression of disappointment.

Allen was a 13-year-old boy brought to me by his mother. She had custody of him and his 8-year-old sister following her divorce from their father. Allen was having problems at school and at home. In addition, his mother expressed frustration over his unwillingness to do his chores. "He just will not listen. I have to tell him four times to get him to put out the garbage!," his mother assured me.

When I saw Allen later, I said, "Allen, your mom tells me that you won't help her around the house." "Oh, but I do!" he insisted. "How?" I asked. "I put out the garbage," he informed me. I challenged him with "Sure you do—after she has told you to four times!" "But, Doctor, she doesn't mean it the first three times!" he said in all seriousness. The scene played out in my mind: "Allen, this is the fourth time I've told you and now I mean business," his mom would say, understandably frustrated as well as angry. Somehow or other Allen's mother had unwittingly suggested to her son that most of the time she didn't "mean business."

2. *Determine whether you are willing to carry out the consequences before threatening your adolescent with them.* Enforcing rules is hard work and not much fun, particularly when the enforcee is someone that the enforcer loves. Sanctions imposed in the heat of anger tend to be tougher than those imposed upon reflection. Having imposed severe sanctions in anger, parents subsequently discover that more than one person is being punished. As one mother told me after her daughter had arrived home very late one night,

I was angry, but mostly I was scared. When Angela finally came home 1 hour late, I was relieved to see that she wasn't dead. But I was furious over her disregard for our feelings, and I grounded her for 6 weeks. Let me tell you, Doctor, those 6 weeks were harder on me than on her. But I stuck to my guns. Six weeks finally passed. I believe I could have accomplished the same lesson in 1 week. But I was determined to carry out the sentence. Angela and I both learned a good lesson.

The question isn't how much can they tolerate, but how much can you? Once imposed, the sentence must be served if there is going to be credibility. Parents more frequently give time off for good behavior for their own benefit than for their child's. But this sends a bad message to their child. It suggests that the parents don't mean what they say. It also allows parents to get off the hook and continue to hand out excessive punishment that has little meaning or predictability. It is helpful to impose sanctions early after an event so that there is a connection between the behavior and the consequences, but calm down first. Sleep on it, then follow up!

3. *The punishment should fit the crime.* When parents are meting out punishment, they should be sure the punishment is appropriate for the rule broken, not as in the following example:

Sammie had been having problems at school, and his parents had brought him to me for evaluation. During one session, he told me that he was getting his driver's license the next day. "You don't seem real excited about it," I observed. "Yeah, my parents are more excited about it than I am. Now they've got something to take away from me. I'm failing Spanish at school, and they said that unless I get a B, they are going to take away my driver's permit," he said with some despair. "What is the connection between driving a car and Spanish?" I asked. He shrugged his shoulders and suggested, "Maybe they think I will get stopped by a Hispanic cop!"

In some ways Sammie was right. Suspending the driving privilege is high on the parental list of potential punishments. The driving privilege is almost a rite of passage for the young adolescent. Even more important is the symbolism of the driving privilege. It suggests the attainment of adulthood. The loss of the driving privilege represents a banishment from adulthood. Failing grades in school should certainly merit some kind of parental response, but there should be a correlation of privilege and responsibility. Perhaps the privilege of driving could be withdrawn as a consequence to Sammie's not meeting his scholastic responsibilities. I would prefer that some other privilege be used. I believe the privilege of driving should be firmly dependent upon safe driving.

Shifting Rules to Your Adolescent

Understanding That, Ultimately, They Must Set Their Own Limits

As I mention in several places throughout this book, one of the main objectives of parenthood is to guide adolescents toward autonomy. Soon they must become young adults who are capable of protecting and setting limits for themselves. Perhaps at this point they still cannot support themselves financially, but there are personal developments going on during young adulthood that will seriously influence their ability to take care of themselves.

Eventually, most parents realize that their adolescents must ultimately set their own limits. This realization is developed gradually through the frustrations parents experience as they try to both protect their young and prepare them to face danger on their own. The adolescent years are filled with risks. Parents can only hope that they have prepared their offspring to take care of themselves. Parents can identify the dangers adolescents face and the behaviors that put them at risk precisely because they too have faced those dangers and confronted many of those problems. They can share some of their solutions with their adolescents, but ought not to demand that these young people become a mirror image of themselves. If the relationship between parents and child is good, most children will try to grow up and be like their parents—unless they believe they are being forced to do so.

Giving Adolescents a Glimpse Into Their Future

I have found it helpful to direct the maturing adolescent's attention toward the ultimate objects of his or her future responsibility: a spouse or partner, possible children, and aging parents. Each day, bright and attractive young people lose their lives. The tragedy is compounded by not only the life that is lost but also those that now will never be. Whatever limits parents set, they must serve the purpose of moving their children toward fulfillment of their future responsibilities. It is useful to pose the challenge in these very words, because adolescents have begun to grasp abstract ideas. These will be intriguing ideas to adolescents, because they point to their future and they define people they have already begun to think about.

Without realizing it, parental rules and limits sound as if they are imposed to make parents' lives better. If adolescents order their lives so that they constantly strive to do whatever is best for their future dependents, parents' lives—and their's—would be better and more successful. Think about it! We don't want them to do what is best for us, but what is best for their future. They owe us very little. They owe their future family much.

For example, I would ask these questions to the maturing adolescent: What will it be like having you for a father? for a mother? for a husband? for a wife? Important people in your life are awaiting you out there in the future. Are you meeting your responsibilities to your son? What can he expect from you? Will your daughter have an educated mother? Will your child have a father who can support her and her mother? Are you meeting your responsibilities to your children? Are you really going to give them a chance to live? Or are you going to risk it all in a moment of irresponsibility?

I tell them that what they think of as their life is not theirs, at least not entirely. Others have a stake in it. Others hope they are taking good care of it.

When You Think Your Adolescent Is Truly Out of Control

Parents usually expect some difficult behavior from their adolescents, but at times, parents feel that they are facing more than the usual difficulties and that their adolescent is out of control. How can a parent tell if this is really the case or if he or she is simply tired of the struggle? Most parents can come up with answers that better fit their particular situation than can the experts. If parents will ask themselves the following few questions, they might come up with some answers:

Do we really have a problem?   Is our child "out of control," or is it that sometimes he or she is either slow to respond or refuses to do whatever we tell him or her to do?

Children should be obedient and respectful; these two should not be confused. The chances are that children are going to disobey their parents on occasion for various reasons. That does not necessarily indicate disrespect. Most children hold their parents in high regard. It is because of their respect for their parents that adolescent struggles are sometimes difficult and frightening. Most adolescents have an exaggerated view of their parents' qualities, even to the detriment of their own sense of worth when measured against their parents.

I have seen children who were literally "beyond parental control." For these children, it isn't simply a matter of their talking back or failing to do what their parents ask. Seriously mentally ill adolescents can present with a loss of control; when this occurs, it is usually obvious that something is seriously wrong. The mentally ill adolescent frequently demonstrates a broad range of behavior that goes far beyond refusal to obey parental directives.

And there are still other adolescents who do unacceptable things but who are not mentally ill. They tend to make the same mistakes over and over, never seeming to profit by those mistakes. They try to shift blame to others and have difficulty in accepting responsibility for their actions. They have little concern for others and have trouble postponing immediate gratification for future reward. These qualities are the manifestations of emotional immaturity.

Any adolescent will demonstrate some degree of unattractive qualities from time to time in his or her struggle toward adulthood. The question for parents is the degree of their presence and the duration of their continuance.

Are we trying hard enough?   How much is hard enough? Well, that depends upon the adolescent and parents who are involved.

Some youngsters are much easier to live with and rear than others. Some parents are able to overlook what they think of as minor transgressions in their child, whereas others are more demanding. Think about whether you are fighting some unnecessary battles.

Is it possible that you are being rougher on yourself than is necessary? Perhaps. The fact that you are reading this book suggests that you have more than a casual interest in trying to understand your adolescent, which signifies that you are most likely a conscientious parent. Most conscientious parents believe that there is but one parental sin: not doing enough. I believe that there is another: doing too much.

Are we working together?

> Mrs. L. was quite angry when she said, "Francesca refuses to come in on time. She never cleans her room. She talks back. She's 15 years old and thinks she is 21. And good ol' Harry here leaves all the discipline to me." At that point, "good ol' Harry" gave his wife a cold stare and said, "My wife is on Francesca's back constantly!" Mrs. L. responded, "Well, if you would help out, I wouldn't have to do it all." Harry then retorted, "If I were to do 50%, Francesca would end up getting 150% of our attention."

It was obvious that these folks had some serious differences in their philosophies of child rearing. Francesca was aware of the conflicting positions and used them to her advantage. Mr. and Mrs. L. had other differences between them, but it was in the area of limit setting that their differences especially manifested themselves. They were not together in their expectations for Francesca. In point of fact, they were not together in their relationship with each other. For limit setting to work, it is imperative for parents to be united. Even when parents are united, children will try to work one against the other. In the above case, limit setting failed repeatedly. Francesca was continuously depressed about her parents' disharmony, and both parents felt like failures.

What are we trying to accomplish? The issue you must address now is, How ready is our child? What still needs to be done?

The following questions will serve as a means for checking up on your child's progress toward adult functioning:

✦ How well does your child function at this point in life?
✦ How well does your child get along with the family? Does he or she feel loved and accepted by the family, and does he or she get along with the family most of the time?
✦ How well does your child get along with friends? Does he or she have at least one good friend?
✦ How well does your child get along in school? (His or her future productivity in the workplace will bear a direct relationship with his or her productivity at school.)

How have we done so far in raising our child?   Ask yourself what qualities you have been trying to instill in your child. There are many traits that serve us well in life. We can get by without some of them, but trying to get by without others will cause trouble. What are these essential qualities?

The following is a short list of qualities that I judge to be important. Each parent should add to or substitute items on this list based on what he or she judges to be important.

1. *Honesty.* How honest is your adolescent? I don't mean has he or she never done anything dishonest, but whether he or she is generally honest in dealings with family and friends. Or does he or she think there is nothing wrong with stealing?

2. *Truthfulness.* For the most part, is your adolescent truthful? Most children might tell a lie at some time or another, especially if compelled to. But can you depend upon their word most of the time? Or does your adolescent say there is nothing wrong with lying? The above two qualities are similar in that truthfulness is honesty of word and honesty is truthfulness of actions.

3. *Industry.* Knowing how and being willing to work is a critical aspect of human character. A father once told me that my patient—his son—was lazy and would not work. He later told me that the boy would spend hours in the hot sun, sanding, smoothing, and polishing his surfboard. "I thought you said he

was lazy and wouldn't work?," I asked. "Oh sure, he'll do that. But that doesn't count. That's something he likes doing!," his father retorted.

Even though this boy did not do the things his father thought of as work, he did show industry and perseverance when it came to an activity he did enjoy. His "laziness" had to do with his not getting the kind of grades his father demanded. Poor grades were his way of saying "you can't make me, so there!" He probably would have given up his surfboard if his father had demanded that he "spend hours in the hot sun sanding, smoothing, and polishing his surfboard."

4. *Compassion.* This quality puts us in touch with our fellow human beings. To possess it we must care about others—not instead of ourselves, but in addition to ourselves. Do you see signs of compassion developing in your child? I don't mean does he or she insist that someone else have the last piece of chocolate cake; rather, how does he or she feel about big kids beating up little kids? Does your child laugh at the suffering of others? Does he or she care about others, even though at times you might feel those "others" are the wrong others? Without this capacity, your child will struggle in this world.

5. *A sense of right and wrong.* Even before becoming an adolescent, most children have more than a mere understanding of what is right and wrong, good or evil, just or unjust. Just let a brother or sister take an unfair advantage, and he or she will receive a dissertation on the miscarriage of justice by a younger sibling. Adolescents possess more than a knowledge of what is right and what is wrong; they have an appreciation of right. They have a clear understanding of how they want to be treated as well as an understanding of how they should treat others. The question is not whether in fact they always do the right thing but how they feel about right and wrong. In evaluating your child's growth and development toward a life characterized by good moral standards, you must not only study his or her behavior but also try to learn how he or she feels about that behavior.

All adolescents at some time or another will do the wrong thing, and after having had time to reflect on their behavior, they do what you and I do: they feel bad about it! The saving grace lies in one's capacity to feel guilt. Guilt is one of our most uncomfortable affects and serves as a deterrent to dishonorable behavior. Most of us strive to avoid behaviors that lead to feelings of guilt, much to the benefit of others around us. I worry about the adolescent who can do evil things and feel no guilt. He or she knows the difference between good and evil in an intellectual way but lacks an appreciation of good.

The foregoing qualities are crucial to a child's ultimate ability to live in this world. The presence of these essential qualities, although not yet fully and firmly in place in their growing child, should help parents understand how well they have done so far.

What else do we need to do as parents? Recognize the enormous influence you have had on the development of your children. That influence continues. Society expects you to have a set of ideals and values by which you conduct your life and then to inform your children of those values in word and deed. If your beliefs and values have been elaborated with a sense of self-improvement and a movement toward your own personal growth and development, they will be worth emulating. Of course, the maxim that "the best laid plans of mice and men often go astray" might become reality. I have seen good parents give it their best shot and still miss the mark. But I have been impressed with the wisdom parents develop in the process of creating and rearing their children.

Conclusion

A word of caution to parents as they examine their children and as they examine themselves. I have found no perfect children. Perfection cannot be given to a child by his or her parents because it is a condition not known in parents. We cannot give that which we do not possess. For the most part, parents do a good job. Some do better. Some do less well. Parents are human beings who possess strengths and weaknesses. They struggle to do the best they can with what they possess, just as your parents did and as your children will do.

Who Are Adolescents?

Chapter 5

Normality and Adolescence

*T*here is something contradictory about expecting normality during adolescence. Many adults believe that adolescence is a disease that can be cured only by time and good fortune. For many years, psychiatrists believed that all adolescents went through considerable turmoil and upheaval on their passage from childhood to adulthood. There was a suggestion that not only was this psychological chaos always present, but that it somehow helped and should be seen as normal. Certainly all the adolescents we saw were going through turmoil, but we weren't seeing normal adolescents. We now know that turmoil is not always present, that it isn't necessarily helpful, and that it doesn't make for a better adult. Of course adolescence is a bumpy ride in some ways. It represents a disruption of what has been until then a rather peaceful journey.

Although the onset of adolescence brings special challenges, it seldom disables an otherwise well-adjusted adolescent. Most adolescents manage to matriculate into and graduate from adolescence without becoming abnormal. In fact, adolescence gets "bad press" in that the average adolescent is less newsworthy than his or her outrageous fellow.

By the time a child reaches adolescence, the family will have elaborated a style of operation and a rather well-defined code of behavior that will be acceptable within the family as well as outside the family or home. And the family will have developed opinions about what to expect from "normal" adolescents. Some of the things adolescents do fly in the face of what is considered normal.

They are not really outrageously abnormal, just "not normal." Most of the not-normal behavior is not necessarily dangerous or destructive. Some behavior is mostly silly. Some behavior is perplexing. Most is merely frustrating. To their elders, that is. That might be why these behaviors happen in the first place. But they have a way of causing parents some anxiety and deliberation of the question, "Is it normal?"

Elsewhere in this book, I describe a young man who appeared in my office with orange hair standing spike-like in a narrow band extending from the front of his head to the rear and flanked on either side by cleanly shaven scalp. His clothing, although not orange, nevertheless had a certain flair for drawing attention. His attire was, fortunately, an exaggeration of ordinary adolescent dress. His psychological state was such that he very much needed to be seen. He was lonely and unhappy, he was having a very difficult time in finding purpose and meaning in his life, and he had a very poor image of himself. He was not a normal adolescent but was struggling with some of the same ordinary adjustments that normal adolescents must face.

Even normal adolescents "rebel" in their dress, their music, and their entertainment, at least partly because this behavior upsets adults. But they also go through role rehearsals as they try to flesh out their budding identities. Moreover, there is a compunction to be correct, that is, correct in the eyes of other adolescents. They absolutely must like the "right" music, wear the "right" clothes, see the "right" movies, and say the "right" thing.

In some ways, we never outgrow the desire to have the approval of our peers. We value what others think of us. But with maturity, "approval" becomes less tyrannizing.

Preadolescence

Preadolescents are in many ways decent and civilized individuals who more often than not will do as they are told. They are ordinarily courteous, respectful, loving, kind, and even prudish in behavior. Freud (1935) described the school age as a period of latency. What has been bubbling away in the psychological development of the young child seems to enter a rather quiescent period that allows the child's psychic energies to be directed toward social and educational endeavors. Whatever the reasons or explanations, juveniles are less frightening than their older siblings.

However, 12-year-old children believe life begins at age 13, and they begin to prepare themselves in anticipation of new rights, privileges, and *freedom*. They begin to watch 13- and 14-year-old adolescents and to make discreet inquiries about how to be an adolescent. They have already learned how to amplify their music and to select only music that will be less than appealing to adults. As a preadolescent, they begin to watch for solid evidence of impending adulthood. They contemplate new behaviors and revel in their prospect.

Defining Normality in Adolescents

In contemplating what is normal and abnormal adolescent behavior, it might help to define the word *normal*. I would like to suggest that *normal adolescent behavior* is that which falls within a range of conduct demonstrated by the average adolescent. What the average adolescent does might not necessarily be proper as viewed by adults. However, I would like to avoid suggesting that normal means proper or good; instead, I emphasize that it only means that it is the norm for that particular group, what is within normal limits. Let me mention an additional caveat: in determining what are normal adolescent behaviors, keep in mind that change is the only constant in the adolescent process.

Offer Studies

Offer and Offer (1975) reported on a long-term study of a group of adolescent males begun in 1962. The work of the Offers has given us a better understanding of the adolescent and the adolescent process.

For the purposes of their study, they selected a group of high school students from two suburban high schools. They eliminated, by psychological testing and psychiatric examination, those students who appeared poorly adjusted and, at the other end of the spectrum, those who appeared extremely well adjusted. The students who fell in the middle of these extremes were designated as the modal group, because it represented the most typical of the larger group. It was this particular group that the Offers followed over the next three decades.

Using the Offer Self-Image Questionnaire, they set out to determine what constitutes normal behavior or mental health in adolescents. Groups of 200–500 adolescents were compared in age groups 13–15 and 16–19 for the 1960s, 1970s, and 1980s.

Offer et al. (1989) reported on data showing that most adolescents function well, enjoy life, and are happy with themselves most of the time. They lack major problems with their body image, and sexuality is not a major problem in their image of themselves. As Offer and his co-workers urged, it is important to understand individual adolescents as they mature.

Adolescents' Behavior Changes Continually

Early adolescence can be sufficiently stressful to create problems. It is not unheard of for adolescents to be cantankerous or to suddenly burst into tears for no apparent reason. They are moody and can descend into the depths of despair in a twinkling, only to bounce right back after one phone call. Dissatisfaction with their bodies and the changes occurring therein is more than offset by the pleasure they feel in acquiring adult status. And they begin to think differently with the onset of a capacity for abstract thinking (see discussion in Chapter 6).

In some ways, adolescents become insufferable with some of their ideas, but in other ways, their evolution toward maturity is a joy to behold and experience. Parents are frequently flabbergasted by an act of thoughtfulness and consideration worthy of the best of maturity and then, conversely, are outraged by certain behavior. Gaining comfort and rejuvenation at a less responsible level, their child once again lurches forward, much to the fragile gratitude of parents and family.

Although trying and frightening at times, average adolescents are also fun. They are funny too. But their humor lacks the symbolism and double entendre of adult humor. There remains an element of juvenile humor with its concreteness. Furthermore, to an extent, adolescent humor contains a larger portion of incompletely disguised hostility. They revel in the "cut-down."

Normal Adolescent Behaviors

Many years ago, I wrote a pamphlet for the South Carolina Mental Health Association at their request and attempted to categorize a variety of behaviors as either normal or abnormal (reproduced in Table 5–1). It was a simplistic declaration, but therein lay its strength and its weakness. In reading it, one must be cautious about categorizing behaviors and suggesting that adolescents should be seen as "within normal limits" rather than as "normal." In addition, I remind the reader that the journey toward adulthood is marked by a chameleon-like quality and by a longing for the privileges of adulthood, as well as the comfort and protection of adolescenthood. What might be normal at age 13 might be less so at age 19.

1. Responsibility for schoolwork. If you have a adolescent who goes to his or her "job" each day (willingly or otherwise), comes home, and prepares himself or herself for the next day on the "job," and then on "payday" brings home a nice "paycheck," you are privileged to be in the company of someone who is mastering one of the most important aspects of maturity, one that is learning how to postpone immediate gratification for future reward. You are also looking at a very desirable future employee.

Adults also go to "school" each day where they do their work and bring home a "report card" at the end of each "marking period." It is signed by an employer rather than a teacher. But an adolescent's report card and an adult's paycheck speak to the external rewards of their endeavors. They indicate how well each is doing his or her job.

Not all adolescents have a high intelligence quotient (IQ) and are able to earn high grades. Similarly, not all adults are able to earn high wages. What might matter more than straight As or big bucks is what is accomplished at school or on the job. I've seen adolescents earn respectable grades without a high IQ. What they had

Table 5–1.   Classification of adolescent behaviors as normal and abnormal

Normal	Abnormal
1. Assumes complete responsibility for schoolwork.	Allows parents to do all the worrying about schoolwork.
2. Identifies with the same-gender parent.	Identifies with opposite-gender parent.
3. Profits by mistakes.	Makes same mistakes again and again.
4. Resents unreasonable rules and verbally expresses resentment.	Resents any rule and expresses resentment of all rules. Alternatively, never breaks or expresses resentment of any rule.
5. Is at times inconsiderate of others, especially brothers and sisters; is at times intensely loyal and considerate of others.	Is never considerate of others; has little or no loyalty to friends.
6. Shows loosening of ties with family and increasing interest in friends.	Has little interest in friends; won't cut apron-strings.
7. Is able to show genuine remorse for misdeeds.	Shows little or no remorse for misdeeds; tends to blame others for them.
8. Is able to show a variety of emotions, including anger, resentment, and jealousy.	Shows either no emotion or only "nice" emotions.
9. Exhibits a moderate amount of untidiness mixed with a moderate amount of neatness.	Is excessively neat and punctual and shows excessive propriety.
10. Looks and acts like an average adolescent.	Is overly conforming to parental wishes in dress and behavior.
11. Is fairly confident that parents love him or her and approve of him or her as a person. Has self-respect.	Feels unloved and unliked as a person. Feels that parents are ashamed of him or her. Has little regard for himself or herself.
12. Causes concern in the older generation.	Causes concern in the older generation.

was a modest IQ and a terrific sense of "I will!" I have observed the same blend of ability and desire in adults.

The following example illustrates how parents sometimes do not allow their adolescent to accept full responsibility for his or her schoolwork:

> The parents of a 16-year-old boy asked me to evaluate their son. He was bright, talented, and articulate, but he was failing at school. "We're afraid he won't be able to get into college with the kind of grades he has earned," his parents confided to me. "We've done everything we know how to motivate him," they assured me. They were both college graduates, socially prominent, popular, well-to-do, and worried to death about their son's future. When I saw their son later, I put the question to him, "How do you expect to get into college with such disgraceful grades?" He smiled, put his hands behind his head, and said, "Doctor, my mother and father are so uptight about my education, I think they'll figure out something!" And they did!

Some adolescents do poorly in school because their lives are chaotic. Some are not bright. But at least some have come to believe that it is their mother's and father's responsibility to cajole, plead, threaten, or beg them to do better.

2. Gender identification. Most boys want to be like Dad, and most girls want to grow up and be like Mom. For one reason or another, the process of gender identity might go awry. (See Chapter 6 for a more detailed discussion.)

Each of us was assigned at birth to either the male or female gender. Each of us understands the expectation that one day we will be a man or one day we will be a woman. Early in life, a process of differentiation begins as we assume more and more of the attributes of our assigned gender. At adolescence, the process accelerates. The adolescent girl who has spent her childhood seeing her mother abused and degraded is liable to have grave doubts about the joy of becoming a woman. If all the power in her family has rested in the hands of her father and has been used to degrade women, she might determine that it is better to be a man and find herself struggling with gender confusion. Similarly, the male is going to be influenced by the risk-benefit ratio of becoming a male by what he has observed in his process of identification with his father.

3. Learning by mistakes.   Most people learn from their mistakes. They confront problems in their lives and attempt to solve them, then develop strategies to cope with similar problems if confronted again. This ability to learn from mistakes is an important quality in emotionally mature adults. Parents who do not allow their adolescent to learn from his or her mistakes are taking away an opportunity for their child to mature, as in the following example:

> A 16-year-old boy wrecked his automobile through reckless driving. His loving parents were grateful that he wasn't hurt and gave him a new car. When their son wrecked that car, too, they again replaced it with another. When I saw this boy, he was driving his fourth new car. He was depressed. He wondered why his parents kept giving him his own automobile. So did I!

4. Reaction to rules.   Reasonable rules are more easily obeyed and therefore more easily enforced. But don't expect adolescents not to complain about rules; they should be allowed to complain. But should they be allowed to break the rules? Of course not!

Adolescents must learn how to express resentment they feel, including expressing resentment to their parents. It's easier to learn how to do this with someone who loves them; resentment can be expressed with fervor and feeling but without obscenities. The statement, "It's alright to express your resentment to me, but I will not tolerate your demeaning me and I'll not tolerate the demeaning of you—not even by you," clearly states parental limits.

Too frequently, adolescents who never express resentment or break any rules are thought of as "good" adolescents. Many are. But some are terrified that they won't be loved if they do anything wrong. That's not normal and not healthy, as in the following example:

> A young adolescent was brought to me because he was failing in school, wetting his bed, and very unpopular with other adolescents. He was otherwise the perfect adolescent: clean, neat, cour-

teous, punctual, kind, considerate, and respectful toward adults.

This boy's mother was a model parent. She too was clean, neat, courteous, punctual, kind, considerate, and very proper. After 6 months of her son's being in treatment, the mother came to me and said, "He's worse!" I inquired about how he was worse. "He's cheeky. He talks back to me," she replied. I wasn't surprised. Her son had begun to feel better about his family and to believe that perhaps they did love him. He felt that he could tell them things that previously he had hidden from them for fear they would exile him. He was a boy who had been terrified that, unless he were perfect, his family would abandon him. When his mother came to understand this, she rejoiced that her son was a much happier boy. She also told me that he was doing better in school, was no longer wetting his bed, and was developing relationships with other adolescents.

5. Being considerate. It is "normal" for the adolescent to be inconsiderate at times. It is "normal" for adolescents to be jealous and inconsiderate of brothers and sisters. Siblings really are competitors for the attention and affection of parents. It is desirable to want them to love one another, play nicely with one another, and stand up for and not be jealous of one another.

On the other hand, the adolescent can be fiercely loyal and considerate of others and get into trouble with parents if the "others" he or she is being loyal to are, in the parents' eyes, the wrong type of people. Parents agonize over this issue when their adolescent defends another adolescent who is always in trouble. "But Dad, you always told me to never kick someone who is down and out. You always told me to give people another chance!" These are the times we need to dig deeply into our store of wisdom.

It's normal for parents to struggle around such issues. It's normal for the adolescent to be considerate of the "wrong" people. What is not normal or healthy is an adolescent who has no compassion or consideration for anyone other than himself or herself. Perhaps it's better for an adolescent to be loyal to people the parents do not like than to feel loyalty to no one!

6. Loosening ties with family. It is normal for adolescents to begin loosening ties with their family during their teenage years. At the same time, adolescents are spending more and more time with friends. It is abnormal when adolescents have no friends and cling unduly to the family. (See further discussion of leaving home in Chapter 10.)

7. Remorse shown, remorse felt.   It is normal for the adolescent to be able to feel genuine remorse for his or her misdeeds. However, failing to *show* remorse is not always proof of its absence. An adolescent boy's refusal to tell his sister that he is sorry he hit her doesn't necessarily prove that he is heartless. Later, when his anger subsides, he will most likely feel bad about what he did. In judging a developing and yet incomplete adolescent, bear in mind that remorse can be felt even when it is not shown.

By the time a child reaches adolescence, he or she knows the difference between right and wrong or good and bad. The overwhelming majority of adolescents are decent human beings who feel bad when they do bad things—if not immediately, at least later. What has always frightened me are the older adolescents who have failed to acquire a conscience. They feel no remorse or guilt.

8. Emotions felt, emotions expressed.   It is human nature for people to experience a wide variety of emotions, even those others think are unacceptable. It is not normal or healthy for an adolescent to show no emotions. It is almost as bad as showing only "nice" emotions.

What people do with their feelings is critical to their existence with others. If adolescents are to be understood by their families, they must be able—and willing—to communicate their feelings. Young children tend to act out their feelings behaviorally. Adolescents must learn how to express feelings not only in deed but also in word. It is far better for a brother to tell his sister about his anger than to hit her. It is far better for an adolescent girl to tell her mother that she is angry with her and why, rather than stuff her anger down deep inside, thereby misleading her mother to believe that everything is okay. It is far better for an adolescent boy to tell someone how depressed he is than for him to express that message in a suicide attempt.

Anger, jealousy, fear, and sadness are unpleasant emotions. But family life is supposed to prepare individuals for managing themselves in adversity as well as in joy. It is within the context of the family that people learn to fight fairly—not by abusing or degrading one another, but by vigorously portraying their point of view in pursuit of mutual understanding. In the family, all individuals learn to reveal their wounds and to seek its love, sympathy, empathy, and support. Adolescents must learn that their feelings are manifestations of their membership in the human race.

It is important for adults to legitimize the presence of feelings not only in their adolescents but also in themselves. If adults cannot come to terms with their own feelings and their legitimacy, they will convey to their children a sense that they do not possess them or that they have only "nice" feelings. Adolescents who see parents who are never angry, jealous, sad, or frightened will try to hide their feelings too. They will come to believe that "there is something wrong with me. I am bad. Mother and Father have only nice emotions. If they ever find out how rotten I am inside, they'll send me away."

9. Tidiness and untidiness. It's normal to see untidiness in adolescents. Some of that is an attempt to be like their friends. Some of it is a way of being "cool" and conveying a sense of nonchalance. Some of it is a way of proving that they are not conformists.

Heaven forbid that I suggest that neatness, punctuality, and promptness be thought of as abnormal or unhealthy. But in excess, it might well suggest an adolescent who is overly constricted. Excessive neatness is seldom a consequence of parental demand. It concerns me if it is present with other personal constrictions to the point of jeopardizing an adolescent's relationship with his or her family and friends.

10. Looks like an adolescent. It's normal for an adolescent to look like other adolescents. Styles being what they are, I dare not define the proper costume currently accepted by the adolescent, as it will change before this book is printed. Also, it is not normal for the adolescent to dress the way I dress. Three-piece suits are not their forte.

11. Feels loved.   Most adolescents believe that their parents love them and approve of them as a person. They have respect for themselves as a consequence. This is normal. Oh, adolescents have moments when they believe that their parents don't love them, but this feeling is transient.

However, it is unhealthy and abnormal for an adolescent to feel truly unloved and unliked as a person. So many of the adolescents who come to me for treatment feel that their parents are ashamed of them. They see themselves as unworthy, have little respect for themselves, and feel no confidence in themselves. (I discuss the adolescent's self-identity in Chapter 6.) Let it suffice to say that feeling loved and accepted is critical to an adolescent's successful development.

12. Worries the older generation.   The abnormal adolescent causes concern in the older generation. The normal adolescent causes concern in the older generation. I'm not sure whether that is a commentary on the adolescent or the older generation!

The foregoing are offered only as generalities and as such are flawed, as are all generalities. They are offered with the recognition that the adolescent developmental process is a dynamic ebb and flow.

Parental Reaction to Teenage Years

What has been a happy and rewarding time for parents erupts into adolescence with all of its implications. Parental anxiety escalates at adolescence, particularly so if it is the first adolescent. As soon as an adolescent's birthday number includes the word *teen,* parents go on the alert. Parents also begin to make discreet inquiries about the oncoming challenge. Parents of preadolescents keep a wary eye on other adolescents and begin to seek the counsel of parents who have already been "initiated."

Most parents are pleased that their adolescent is growing up, and they look forward to the pleasure of seeing their child acquire beauty and strength. These parents are happy, proud, and worried! Strength and beauty have all manner of implications. With that strength comes the capacity to inflict physical hurt on others. With that beauty comes the attention of others, some not very desirable.

Parents Were Once Adolescents

Two of the powerful forces each person must master during adolescence are aggressivity and sexuality. Each person must develop his or her own method of harnessing these forces and directing them into productive and healthy channels. By the time adolescents experience these feelings, they have developed a personality of their own, which greatly influences how they manage these new forces. Their experiences within the family and their genetic heritage help determine how they react. Many adolescents feel overwhelmed by these forces, and with naught but good intentions, bury them deeply inside while assigning nothing but bad feelings to them.

Once adolescents reach adulthood, they have adjusted and gotten on with their lives. Each faced these drives and applied his or her own special brand of management in order to establish healthy control. But, now as parents of an adolescent, they must watch as their adolescent confronts the same challenges. Old wounds begin to ache as parents watch their adolescent struggle. Parents must now attempt to steer their adolescent through these troubled times. Their success will vary depending upon how well they managed their own adolescence, what they have learned since, and how much they have grown personally.

Parents who still find themselves in a desperate situation, with their most intimate human relationship a source of nothing more than pain, and who still have not come to terms with themselves, will have difficulty determining what are normal and adaptive adolescent behaviors. How can they help their adolescent find that which still eludes them? Most parents of adolescents have found meaning and value in their lives, at least to some degree. Those who have become stuck somewhere along the path will do well to recognize the wonderful opportunity occasioned by the flowering of their adolescent while they contemplate their own destiny.

Determining When Something Is Wrong With an Adolescent

My experience with many, many parents has led me to believe that most parents have a fairly good idea about what is right and what is wrong. I believe that most parents possess adequate problem-solving skills and, given the opportunity to use those skills, make the right decision more often than not. Part of the problem clusters around conflicting views of one parent or the other or conflicting views of other family members or important friends. Too often, parents lack faith in their own judgment and seek advice here, there, and everywhere. Trying to decide what is normal (acceptable) and what is abnormal (unacceptable) in their adolescent will require clear communication between parents.

Criteria for Interpreting an Adolescent's Behavior

I think of the normal adolescent as one who functions well in the three principal areas of his or her life. When I am asked to evaluate an adolescent, I inquire about these areas by asking myself three questions:

1. How well is this adolescent getting along with his or her family?
2. How well is this adolescent performing on his or her job?
3. How well is this adolescent functioning in relation to his or her friends?

These questions represent significant aspects of an adolescent's life. Indeed, they represent significant aspects of anyone's life. How well a person does in these three areas of life will tell much about the normalcy of that person's life.

How well is this adolescent getting along with his or her family?   When I see an adolescent who is not getting along with his or her family, I worry. I don't mean the natural disagreements with parents or siblings. Here, I am talking about the serious disruption of a relationship with the family to the extent that it is an ongoing source of pain for the adolescent and the family, a relationship that is as unfulfilling for one as it is for the other. I am talking about a dysfunction that is apparent and obvious.

It is not normal for an adolescent to be unable to get along with his or her family over a prolonged period. Getting along with most family members, most of the time, is the norm. If an adolescent is not getting along well with those who love him or her most, that adolescent is dysfunctional in a major area of life and probably would benefit from counseling. For some adolescents, the dysfunction manifests itself only at home.

Adolescents will become depressed if they feel that they are unloved by those who are supposed to care for them. That depression will be manifested by unremitting sadness or will be disguised as outrageous behavior. But it is not easy for young adolescents to talk about depression. A family that is accustomed to talking about feelings will be in a better position to detect depression in an adolescent. As a matter of fact, the family that is accustomed to talking about feelings will not only detect emotional dysfunction early on, but more likely is doing the very thing that will help prevent dysfunction. For if a family is a "psychological support system designed to sustain its members during periods of adversity," as noted in Chapter 1, it will be alert to the pain of its members and ready to repair.

How well is this adolescent performing on his or her job?
For adolescents, the most honorable occupation is that of student. There is a significant correlation between how well they do at school today and how well they will do tomorrow on the job. The adolescent who is not getting along well at home, but who is doing just fine at school, demonstrates a higher level of competence than those who are not only not getting along well at home but also failing at school. These latter adolescents worry me more. If an adolescent is dysfunctional in two-thirds of his or her life, professional evaluation should be seriously considered.

It is a bit misleading to suggest that an adolescent's life is, or can be, compartmentalized. It is even more misleading to suggest that those compartments won't leak. Each area of dysfunction can spill over into other areas. It is difficult to feel depressed and un-loved at home and yet happily excel at school. Some manage better than others. Observant teachers who see falling grades at school almost always wonder, "What's going on at home?" Observant parents who notice withdrawal and remoteness in their youngster always wonder, "What's going on at school?"

How well is this adolescent functioning in relation to his or her friends?   All three areas of an adolescent's functional devel-opment are important, but his or her ability to make and maintain friends has a way of intruding into the other areas of life. I have seen adolescents who were in ongoing battles with their families and doing poorly in school but widely popular with friends—adults as well as peers. This says something about their ability to survive in a world of other people.

On the other hand, success in school and work and good family relations can bring a degree of happiness. The child who is unable to make a connection with his or her fellow humans faces a lonely life.

Is the adolescent having trouble in all three areas?   The ad-olescent who is not getting along at home, is failing at school, and has found that other adolescents do not like him or her has three strikes against him or her. That adolescent is in need of skilled pro-fessional care.

Throughout my career of working with adolescents, it was this last group that caused me the most concern. These were the ado-lescents I admitted to the hospital. More than a few of these ado-lescents have a mental illness but not all. Temporizing in the treatment of a disintegrating mental illness is inexcusable. With-holding medication from an adolescent who is psychotic is as un-justified as the act of medicating adolescents unnecessarily. When an adolescent's life hangs in the balance, he or she needs highly skilled care, perhaps in an intensive care facility.

There are no simple and absolute measuring sticks for deciding which adolescent needs what. The foregoing considerations were only part of my deliberations in devising proper psychiatric care for adolescents—but an important part.

Working With Troubled Adolescents

Look to the Context of the Family

When I encounter a troubled adolescent, the first thing I look at in order to evaluate and understand that adolescent is how he or she functions in the context of his or her family, for it is there that he or she is being taught autonomy. When a family is meeting its responsibilities to its members, it is functioning properly. When a family is not meeting its responsibilities to its members, both the member and the family are dysfunctional.

I have learned that if I listen only to an adolescent telling me what is going wrong, I almost always hear a list of complaints about the parents and how they are causing the adolescent's problems. If I listen only to the parents, I get a different view: parental views tend to focus on the adolescent as the problem. Although they each have different views, many times both views are right; that is, most families malfunction for more reasons than one.

In Search of a Solution

Even though I can often deduce the cause of many adolescents' problems within the first hour of talking with them, the solution requires many hours. Why? Because although the problem is obvious to me as an outsider, it would be incorrect to assume that it is also obvious to the insiders. Usually, each participant is trying to do the "right" thing. However, the problem is that his or her view of what is right and what is wrong is usually obscured by many forces.

Another barrier to solving problems is the difficulty in deciding the right course of action to take. Most parents, given a choice between doing what is right or what is wrong, will always choose to do the right thing. That's easy! But what is a parent to do when the choice lies between doing what is wrong and what is also wrong? Parents frequently find themselves struggling with choices in which they cannot be assured of a happy solution. Forced to choose between two wrongs, they seek the "rightest wrong" and cross their fingers.

Parents Must Be Unified in Approaching Problems

In elaborating a plan to correct unacceptable behavior or attitudes in their adolescent, parents must clearly communicate their views and truly collaborate in their efforts. Even when each parent brings opposing views, consensus can be pursued and found. Sometimes, mothers know what is more normal for a daughter than a father would and deserve to have some extra points when deliberating the matter. Sometimes, good fathers, who are also loving husbands, are entirely too protective of their daughters and consequently seem too strict in the daughter's view. When two parents differ in their view of what is right and wrong for their adolescent, clear and open communication becomes critical. Such a circumstance presents a great opportunity for a husband and a wife to negotiate a unified position and to strengthen the relationship between them.

This situation also offers one more opportunity for parents to learn something about each other. As they talk about their adolescent, they also are given the opportunity to learn about themselves. One parent might say, "Perhaps I am being too strict, but I'm so afraid that she might get hurt," as he or she tries to protect those he or she loves. Such a circumstance also offers an opportunity to discharge pent up anger and frustration to an unsympathetic spouse. If the relationship between mother and father is an unhappy one, the struggle between them might be deflected, unwisely, onto the adolescents as they deliberate what is normal or abnormal for those adolescents.

The Family as a Source of Healing

So many parents have brought their adolescent to me for evaluation and, at the outset of that evaluation, jokingly suggest, "Gosh, Doctor, you may find that we are the problem!" That declaration was almost always accompanied by nervous laughter and fervent hopes that it was not true. "Nothing would make me happier," is my standard reply. I tell them

> You love this adolescent so much that you are willing to bring him [or her] to me and risk the pain your visit might bring. I hope you

are "the problem" because if you are, I know you will help me make your adolescent well. Adolescents almost always develop their psychological disabilities in the context of their family. When that is so, it is also true that there is where they will be repaired. The human family possesses an enormous recuperative power that can go far in the restoration of function.

In working with adolescents, the family has occupied a central role in all of my treatment (Orvin 1974). I began including families when that was not yet popular. I did so for a very good reason: I needed all the help I could get. Moreover, I suspected that excluding parents from the treatment process would cause justified resentment in the parents and resistance against my efforts. I think it is critically important to co-opt parents into the treatment process from the very beginning.

Although bad things can happen to an adolescent, which have little or nothing to do with his or her family, the family's participation and support are important. When the cause of the problem lies outside of the family, it is not easy to enlist the enthusiastic support of nonrelated "guilty parties."

Conclusion

When individuals contemplate what is normal or abnormal in human behavior, they are seeking a pathway to adaptive and productive living with other human beings. Parents' wish for normal behavior in their adolescents is at least partly prompted by their desire that their adolescents might come to find that harmony in their own lives. As parents examine the progress their adolescents are making toward maturity, they really are evaluating the effectiveness of the family in its mission. If an adolescent is on course and moving toward the normal development of maturity, autonomy, and emancipation, at least one of the family's missions is being met.

Chapter 6

Adolescents' Evolving Personal Identity

Many adults become impatient with adolescents who are trying to "find" themselves. One mother sheepishly confessed,

> I wish he wouldn't even bother with this. At least, I wish he would hurry and get it over with. He mopes around the house, constantly examining himself in the mirror, and he is liable to suddenly blow up in anger or burst into tears. Our friends tell us he is "trying to find himself." My husband says that if our son doesn't get it over with, someone will have to come and try to find us!

In some ways, adolescence is a process of searching and trying to "find" oneself. It is a time of moping but also a time of scintillating joy as the adolescent robes himself or herself in the various possibilities of fame and fortune. The process of "finding" is a venture of role rehearsal, but it is more than choosing a career.

Much of his or her preoccupation lies in the question of "what kind of person am I becoming?"

Adolescents Develop
New Powers of Self-Analysis

Changing From Concrete to Abstract Thinking

Preadolescent children certainly know who they are. Just ask one of them, "Who are you?" and you'll hear, "I'm Jimmy Jones, and I live at 126 Maple Street," or something similar. If we ask Jimmy to tell us what sort of person he is, he might not understand. Abstract thinking and understanding are lacking in younger children. As another example, if one asked an 8- or 9-year-old child, "What do I mean when I say 'People who live in glass houses ought not throw stones?'" he or she would probably respond, "Because you might break the glass."

But something happens just before entrance into adolescence that opens up a whole new world for children. They don't experience a major growth in intelligence, but they do begin to develop a new mental capacity that allows them to see the world differently. What had always been either black or white becomes various shades of gray. What had always been right or wrong now seems less clearly defined. People seem different as well. Some of those who were once thought of as perfect now seem less so. Others who were once seen as all bad now seem to have parts of them that are not all bad. At this point in their mental and emotional life, adolescents begin to develop skills and capacities that allow them to understand their environment and themselves as well as others like and unlike themselves. The power to reason, analyze, and discriminate is developing.

Piaget (1950) spent a lifetime studying the development of intellectual functioning in humans. He described several stages of development in infants, adolescents, young adults, and adults. The highest level of development he termed *formal operations,* which applied to a capacity for a new kind of thinking. Between ages 7 and 11, children think in rather concrete terms but begin to do exciting things mentally and intellectually. A large amount of education is accomplished during these years, but a certain kind of thinking remains to be developed, which is reserved for the next stage. Attainment of formal operations begins around age 11 or 12 and becomes available to adolescents at a very important time in their life. Adolescents begin to understand the hidden message in proverbs such as the one quoted above. As they develop a capacity for abstract thinking, adolescents can contemplate their own thinking. They develop the ability to understand the use of symbols and, consequently, symbolic thinking.

Using New Skills to Form Self-Identity

At this stage, adolescents are able to see themselves as a symbol in that they can figuratively take three steps away, turn, and contemplate themselves in their own mind. They now become interested in viewing themselves through the eyes of others. What do other people think of me? and What sort of a person do I think I am? are questions that send them in pursuit of a personal definition and a sense of personal identity. This is a time for the taking of inventory. From the shelves of their memory, they now count the accumulation of what they have heard about themselves and what they have seen of their worthiness to those who are supposed to know them best.

Erikson (1950) described the central task of adolescence as the consolidation of a firm sense of identity. Failure to do so leads to what Erikson called *role diffusion,* or the inability to develop a firm sense of identity. Adolescents indulge in a variety of role rehearsals as they begin to experiment with what and who they might become. They begin to weave the fabric of their identity in preparation for the assumption of adulthood. They use their newly found mental skills and also draw upon several external sources in the process of self-evaluation as they search for this sense of identity. One of the more important sources of information is the peer group (see discussion of the peer group below).

During its early development, the sense of personal identity is incomplete, vulnerable, and, in some ways, still fragile. Events and circumstances in adolescents' lives take on powerful meanings and can become woven into the fabric of their identity. Experiences occurring at this time can assume exaggerated importance beyond their measure. The same experiences occurring after the consolidation of a sense of self might have little or no effect. For example, strong feelings of affection for a friend of the same gender can be very frightening to the adolescent, leading to questions such as "Am I homosexual?" Not being invited to a certain party might cause an adolescent to feel ugly and unwanted. How people see or think of him or her can provoke great anxiety in the incomplete adolescent.

The process of evolving a sense of personal identity should be a lifelong task in that all individuals should continue to grow. The definition of who a person is expands as that person comes to know more about himself or herself. But it is during adolescence that individuals begin that critical work.

Adolescents See Themselves in the Eyes of Their Peers

How do young adolescents go about the process of elaborating a sense of personal identity? It is true that they use the peer group as a source of information about themselves. The peer group is a social validation experience. But it is overrated! The mention of the words "peer group" strikes terror into the hearts of adolescents' parents. They see the peer group as a band of brigands about to spirit their helpless adolescent away from the protection of home and off to some nefarious fate. Not so.

Social Validation

The peer group is more or less a gathering of awkward contemporaries struggling with the same psychological work. It is an ad hoc group—that is, the membership may change at any moment. The group may drop two members and let two more in. The peer group is a dynamic organization that changes its requirements for membership from time to time. But it is valuable. The peer group's message to the successful applicant is, yes, you wear the right clothes, you listen to the right music, you use the right slang, you say the right things, and so on. Basically, the group is saying, "You are like us; therefore, you are okay." The peer group can bring the joy of acceptance by one's fellow human beings or the pain of repudiation. All of that is helpful for most adolescents, because most adolescents don't need much more than that. But some do. (See discussion below of adolescents with a poor self-image.)

Peer Group Influence Is Transient

The influence of the peer group is transient. Reflect on the brevity of the young adolescent's relationship with the peer group. Compare the time spent with a peer group with the millions of human interactions that an adolescent has had with his or her family up to that point. What makes the peer group seem so critically important is that adolescents are in a process of discovery about themselves, and during this part of self-discovery, how the peer group feels and thinks can be important.

The peer group's influence on the adolescent rises or falls depending upon how the adolescent feels about himself or herself, something that has, for the most part, been determined elsewhere. The adolescent who feels loved and respected by his or her family has less need for approval from other sources. The adolescent who feels unloved and unvalued will seek approval wherever it can be found. The more he or she needs that approval, the higher the price he or she is willing to pay in order to get it.

Many of the adolescents who have come to me needed much, much more than a nice peer group. Most had such a rotten view of themselves that no peer group could ever change their view. Many of them had already decided that they were not worthy of life. Some had already tried to relieve the world of their unworthiness by eliminating themselves. How in the world did these adolescents come to this view of themselves? Did the peer group cause this? Not likely. Can the peer group cure this? Not likely!

Adolescents See Themselves Through Their Parents' Eyes

If it isn't peer groups' influence that causes adolescents to develop a poor view of themselves, then what can? The next place to look is the family.

What Do Adolescents Believe Their Parents Think of Them?

It has always been my standard practice to ask certain questions of my adolescent patients at the outset of the interview. One question is, "What sort of person are you?" I mostly get looks of perplexity, frequently accompanied by shrugged shoulders and upturned palms. Many cannot answer; they do not know the answer because evolving a sense of personal identity is what adolescence is all about. I ask this question, knowing it might not be answered, as a way of introduction to another, very provocative, question: "Well then, suppose I were to ask your father to tell me what sort of person you are. How do you think he would answer my question?"

This is a loaded question! Many adolescent patients respond with a look of bewilderment, shrug their shoulders, turn up their palms in a gesture of helplessness, and reply, "I don't know!" Some stare off into space contemplating my question and then answer, "Well, if you asked my father what sort of person I am, he would tell you that I'm lazy, that I'm stupid, that I'm irresponsible, that I'm rude, that I'm a . . . delinquent!" I listen patiently and carefully. I then say, "If he thinks that's the sort of person you are, tell me how he feels about you." Another look into space, another shrugged shoulder, and two more upturned palms answer me with exquisitely painful eloquence.

I once asked a 15-year-old girl to tell me how her mother would answer my question. She dropped her head, and when she looked up, she was crying. "My mother would tell you that I am a tramp!" she answered. "So, how does she feel about you?" I asked. She shook her head. She couldn't talk. At that point, neither could I! I'm sure that her mother didn't think she was a tramp; at least, she probably didn't mean it when she called her that.

When I ask patients' parents to tell me how they thought their son or daughter had answered the question, "What sort of person do your parents think you are?" I get some interesting answers. For example: "Oh, I think he'd tell you that I'm a fairly good father, Doc." That's an answer to the wrong question! But fathers do worry whether they are being good fathers. In response to the question, other fathers shrug their shoulders, raise their palms in a gesture of helplessness, and reply, "I don't know how he [or she] answered your question." Still others, who didn't like my question, merely glowered at me. The truth was, they didn't like what they thought was the answer. They were afraid of their adolescent's answer.

Think about it! A parent and a child, having lived cheek-by-jowl for at least 13 years, and neither can say what they think of one another or how one feels about the other! What in the world has gone wrong? Poor communication? But they do communicate! They talk about things, about places, and about other people. What they don't talk about is how they feel—how angry they are, how jealous they are, how sad they are, how scared they are, or how they feel about each other.

It's important that parents understand this particular task of identity formation. And even though your adolescent might not be a troubled adolescent, this is a time of questioning by even healthy youngsters. What their parents think of them is important. What is even more important is what they think their parents think of them. Most parents hope their adolescent knows how they feel, but do they really? So strong are the feelings of love that parents have for their children that they sometimes make a critical error and conclude that surely their children "know" how much they love them. I want to suggest that they might hope and even believe that their parents love them, but I doubt that they "know" how their parents feel.

Children who approach adolescence believing that they are loved by their parent or parents bring with them a powerful tool to be used in the elaboration of their sense of personal identity. Most do believe their parents love them and that they are lovable. The important point here is that as they go through the "process of becoming," the way they feel about themselves will bear a close relationship to how the significant people in their lives feel about them. Factored into this is the ability of adolescents' parents to express those feelings clearly and the adolescents' ability to perceive them clearly.

Most adolescents survive the adolescent process without seeking approval elsewhere, mostly because they feel the love and caring of their parents and families. Most adolescents feel good about themselves in a very healthy way. They have had 13 or 14 years of acceptance from those they love and admire. They have had 13 or 14 years of hearing some good things about themselves in addition to some bad things. They have had 13 or 14 years of observing the adults in their life conducting themselves in effective and worthy inter-actions with one another and with other adults. Most adolescents don't desperately need the approval of a peer group—any peer group.

Adolescents With a Poor Self-Image

I worry about adolescents who feel rotten about themselves. These are the adolescents at risk, particularly as they begin to add up the score on themselves. This is what makes the evolution of a sense of personal identity such a painful experience for troubled adoles-cents. Bad feelings about themselves won't be new to adolescents in this situation. Up to this point, they have somehow been able to pretend that they were or would soon become lovable, that magic would make it better, or that "they" would start caring about them. With the arrival of adolescence begins the development of analyti-cal skills and deductive reasoning. Now adolescents have the skills necessary to see what rotten individuals they really are. They keep adding up the score, and it keeps coming out zero.

In addition, as mentioned above, at the beginning stages of ado-lescence, one's ego is only partially developed, which makes the adolescent vulnerable to assaults from outside and within. Once a strong sense of personal identity has been developed, the individual develops a degree of immunity to threats to the ego. What might be very damaging to a 13-year-old person's ego might be much less damaging to a 25-year-old person's ego. But during the early and middle stages of adolescence, much is at stake. And for adolescents who feel unloved, their other source of immunity—the approval of their primary caregivers—is also absent, rendering them even more vulnerable to threats from the outside world.

Seeking Approval Elsewhere

The evolution of a sense of identity, as well as the other tasks of adolescence, constitute psychological growth. Psychological growth is hard and, at times, painful work. Those adolescents who feel unloved, unvalued, and of little concern to those they love may seek relief of the pain through other avenues. The great risks for adolescents come at a time when they are doing difficult psychological work and at a time in their life when they are mobile enough to seek relief outside the family (see further discussion of this issue in Chapter 9).

This is the profile of an adolescent who desperately needs the peer group. But "the" peer group doesn't want "losers!" But there are other peer groups to which these adolescents can apply. There is the drug peer group, the delinquent peer group, the disaffected peer group, and the underachieving peer group. Once an adolescent falls in with the behavior of these alternative peer groups (e.g., by using drugs, becoming delinquent), he or she changes from becoming a nobody that no one wanted to being a somebody who is accepted into a group. And maybe, in a maladaptive way, it is better to be a drug taker than it is to be a nobody.

The great tragedy is that troubled adolescents discover that with a few drinks of alcohol or a few puffs of marijuana, they can temporarily relieve the pain of psychological growth. By using drugs, they avoid psychological growth, thus staying lifelong adolescents. The greater their pain, the greater their need is to relieve it. The more they use substances as a form of relief, the more taking those substances becomes an automatic response to anxiety. Instead of feeling lonely and unloved, these adolescents begin to believe they are popular and lovable. Substance use and abuse become solutions for them. But it is not only drugs that offer this escape. Other maladaptive solutions can be equally destructive. Adolescents can use other forms of risk-taking behavior during this period of uncertainty.

Parents know the dangers of drug and alcohol abuse and the peril of the drug and alcohol abuse peer group. Frantically they may shout, "Don't do that! Leave that group! You will get hurt! You will come to know pain!" However, what the adolescent hears is, "Give that up and go back and be a nobody, a nothing, a zero!" Before parents can ask their adolescent to give up his or her maladaptive behavior, they have to understand that what the adolescent needs first is to feel better about himself or herself. And if an adolescent succeeds in leaving the alternative peer group, he or she may still face rejection by "the" peer group, because they do not want "druggies."

Peer groups serve as stepping stones from the family toward independent living. The adolescent seeking rehabilitation from the drug peer group needs to rework his or her relationship with his or her family because it is there we come to feel good about ourselves, and it is there we will be healed.

It is not a quick fix of a pat on the back. Giving up the alcohol and drugs is the first step, but it won't last if the underlying problem isn't resolved. Alcoholism is more than a drinking problem; it is a sobriety problem. In the person who abuses alcohol or drugs, intoxication brings relief of the pain. With the return of sobriety comes the return of pain and anguish. One must do more than avoid alcohol and drugs; one must scrutinize sobriety, which is where the problem lies.

Conclusion

For the adolescent, "Who am I?" is a question that seeks a judgment as to personal worthiness. The "I" part is more than a summation of physical characteristics; it is to a large extent what one thinks and how one feels, especially about oneself. The work of elaborating a sense of self and of finding an encouraging answer to personal worthiness will allow the adolescent to find a way through these years of uncertainty. Although the adolescent seeks independence with a fervor, even more important is a sense of personal worthiness. By the time the adolescent reaches age 21 or 22, the personality or ego will have reached a degree of maturation that will provide him or her with a degree of immunity against psychological dysfunction.

Today, the process of identity formation is more prolonged than it was many years ago, when people would begin a family in their late teenage years or early 20s. As Collange (1988) observed, many young people are still at home at age 25 or even at age 30. She noted that "in France, three-fourths of the 18 to 25 year olds still live under the parental roof. . . . From the middle ages to today we have added 30 years to the length of life and at least 10 years to the deferring of it."

The evolution of a sense of personal identity is not completed by the end of adolescence. Even adults continue to add to their sense of self. But by the end of adolescence, one's personality structure has become more mature, more solid, and less vulnerable. For the most part, the ego has been consolidated.

Chapter 7

Adolescents' Evolving Sexual Identity

I Want to Be a Man

I am a 13-year-old boy, and I want to be a man. What should I begin doing in order to become a man? People tell me to grow up. Some say, "Act your age!" Others say, "Stop being a child." Everyone tells me what to do, but no one tells me how!

So how do I stop being a child? I want to. I really do. I can see my body changing so I know something is happening. My voice sounds deeper sometimes. But just when I want to say something important or something serious, I squeak! And then everyone laughs.

I have a long black hair growing on my chin. But only one. I have other things growing on my face, but I don't want "hick-eys." My feet get in the way sometimes, and my mother says I'm clumsy. My sister aggravates me, then I barely tap her and she bawls. I really didn't mean to hit her that hard. Sometimes my strength surprises me.

I get strange feelings. Some I like, and some scare me. I get very sad and feel awful sometimes. But then, there are times when I feel wonderful. Sometimes I act silly. But I also get real cranky. I wonder what's going to happen to me.

I used to not like Margy, but now she seems real nice. She sure has changed. I don't mind if my friends see me walking with her now. But sometimes I get some real strange feelings about her. And not only when I'm around her. What in the world would I do if someone found out? Or if she found out?

I Want to Be a Woman

I'm a 13-year-old girl, and I want to be a woman. I want to look like a woman, act like a woman, and have people treat me like a woman. Will I ever get rid of these braces on my teeth? I bet I'd look more like a woman if Mom would let me wear lipstick, mascara, and eye shadow. Maybe I could talk Mom into letting me wear stockings and high-heeled shoes. I can see the changes in my body, and Mom says that I'm already becoming a woman now that I menstruate. It means I can have a baby. Doesn't that mean that I'm a woman?

Boys seem nicer now. Even Jody. He seems to like walking with me now. And his friends don't seem to tease him. What would I do if he asked me for a date? Dad will probably want me to wait until I'm 100 years old—or at least 16!

Hormonal Changes in Adolescents

Thus it begins: boys becoming men and girls becoming women. Each gains the necessary physical capacities to reproduce themselves. The physical changes that take place are part of a process defined as *puberty*. The psychological and social changes are part of the process of adolescence. It is somewhat misleading to suggest these are separate processes because each influences the other.

Hormonal changes begin to take place even before outward evidence of sexual growth. Prepuberty and preadolescence can be detected in children by an increase in tension, clumsiness, and irritability. Once hormonal changes begin to take place, the ebb and flow of hormones propel wondrous feelings through the adolescent's body. An enormous tide of anxiety comes with those feelings, mixed with both pride and embarrassment. The adolescent girl is concerned that her breasts might jiggle—or worse, that they won't. The adolescent boy is terrified that he might have a sudden, spontaneous erection just as the teacher sends him to write at the blackboard. And everyone will shriek with laughter! There is the ongoing fear that someone will find out what they do with themselves when alone.

Although most research we know of on development has been

regarding boys (Offer 1969), the topic of gender differences needs to be discussed.

Changes in Young Males

The preadolescent boy might have begun his growth spurt before puberty, but most will not. At adolescence, boys experience an increase in the size of their genitals. They experience uninvited erections, at times independent of sexual thoughts. Their increase in masturbation can be ascribed more to a relief of inner tension than to adult sexual fantasies.

In preadolescence and early adolescence, boys tend to congregate in all-male groups, shunning females. In response to a need to begin disavowing dependence, they begin to actively oppose the very best of parental intentions. They are noisy and rambunctious and are given to argumentativeness, shouting, and door slamming.

Boys tend to undergo most of their growth between ages 13 and 15, with some not entering their growth spurt until age 18. Much of that growth is initially in arms and legs, so their movements can become clumsy. They look and feel awkward, feelings that can be accompanied by embarrassment and irritability.

The other part of the hormonal surge is manifested in the sprouting of pubic and underarm hair. Production of sperm begins in boys between ages 14 and 16.

Changes in Young Females

Evidence of sexual development occurs earlier in girls than in boys. Girls begin to grow taller sooner than boys, with girls having their growth onset around ages 10 and 11 and reaching their full stature by age 15 or 16. Onset of menses for girls starts between ages 10½ and 15.

The young adolescent female becomes very concerned about her body and is given to much dissatisfaction with what she finds. She tends to compare herself with other girls and finds herself too fat, too short, too tall, too thin, or too whatever. She sees other changes in the shape of her body, some of which are a source of pride or embarrassment. A 17-year-old girl recalled the excitement of discovery of her breasts in these words: "When I was about 12 years old, I awoke one morning lying on my back and gazed down at my chest, and there they were. Not much. But mine, all mine!" Nothing could have been more declarative of her arrival into womanhood.

As with young males, the young female must begin to move away from infantile dependence on her mother and, as a consequence, begins to find fault with her mother. If there is one person she fights with more than her sister, it is her mother. Paradoxically, even though she struggles to deny her dependence on her mother, for the most part, her mother is her model.

Boys her own age are of little interest to the female adolescent because they are so "immature." She compensates by shifting her interests to older males. It is not unusual for the young female to have a crush on an older male teacher or an otherwise unavailable and famous celebrity. Although she involves herself with other girls her own age, she frequently finds one girl with whom she shares confidences. These relationships can be intense. They can be extremely valuable to the developing female because it is here that she finds someone who sees the world through similar eyes, and it is here that she begins to learn what it means to be a woman.

Gender Identity Development

For many years, I have lectured that evolving sexual identity is really the evolution of gender identity. During adolescence, young people begin to develop the behavior, attitudes, and characteristics of the gender to which they were assigned at birth. *Gender identity* is much more descriptive of what takes place in the process of adolescence than that of sexual identity. Sexual function is a part of gender identity. Gender is much broader in its implications and speaks more clearly about what it means to be a woman or to be a man.

Adolescents Need Same-Gender Model

The grand scheme of nature is to equip each household with a working model of each gender: one mother and one father. Children who are able to develop a close relationship with an adult male and an adult female in their daily environment are fortunate.

But not all children are so blessed. Death, divorce, or estrangement can deprive children of the luxury of these two parental models. And it is difficult for one parent to take on the role of the other, absent parent. In the case of divorced parents, it is most helpful if the parents can maintain a clear understanding of the psychological needs of their child or children and permit and encourage a positive psychological connection with either the departed parent or provide a satisfactory substitute role model for them (e.g., a grandfather, uncle, male coach, or male teacher for a boy; a grandmother, aunt, female coach, or female teacher for a girl). Of course, very effective modeling can be done by stepmothers and stepfathers.

Given two fundamental conditions, a child will try to grow up and become "just like Dad" or "just like Mom." The first of these two conditions is that the mother or father be able and willing to communicate his or her love to the child. This is different from simply loving a child—that is a given. Parental love is a biological function. It does not require effort to initiate it. What is not a biological given is the capacity to communicate one's love, even parental love. The second requirement for the child's identification with the parent of the same gender is that the parent be available; if not the biological parent, then a parent substitute.

Although children look to the parent of the same gender for their gender identity, they draw other aspects of the personalities of both parents. As the child grows, he or she incorporates bits and pieces of the parents into his or her developing personality.

Explicit modeling of gender-specific behaviors. Emerging adolescents need working models whereby they may measure and monitor their movement toward gender maturity. To bake a cake, one needs a recipe. To build a sailboat, one needs a blueprint. How does one follow a pattern that is unavailable? Adolescent boys need to know how men behave, think, feel, and perhaps smell, and adolescent girls need to know the same about women. Both will benefit enormously by living in close proximity to an adult model of the same gender. Without even trying, fathers teach their sons, and mothers teach their daughters.

Implicit lessons about gender-specific behaviors. So many of the lessons parents teach have little do with what they say. The critical lessons are not what they say, but what they do. Children don't always listen, but they're almost always watching! For example, fathers usually talk with their sons about what it means to be a man and how men should treat women. But even the noblest words will fall on deaf ears if that son has seen a lifetime of neglect or abuse of his mother by his father. As another example, how does a 13-year-old girl define her genderhood and her relations with the opposite gender if her mother does naught but ridicule the child's father?

By the time children reach adolescence, most have observed a male-female relationship in operation through most of their years. Even when the family has been split by divorce, they have seen their mother and father either living together or apart. What they have heard and observed from parents will affect their view of what it means to be a woman or what it means to be a man.

Homosexuality

The question of gender identity is closely bound to sexuality. However, they are different in significant ways. There are only two genders: male and female. But sexuality has to do with more than reproduction. There is an inner tension in all people that seeks release through sexual function.

One's choice of sexual object is influenced by many things, some of which are unconscious. When the object of one's sexual striving is a member of the same gender, it is described as *homosexual* in the male and *lesbian* in the female. Traditionally, the process of object selection has been understood as being primarily a personal choice or caused by unconscious psychological determination. Current research presents some evidence that the process of object selection is at least partly determined by genetics (Bailey and Pillard 1991).

The young adolescent might be attracted to a member of the same gender with or without a sexual component. Although the object of one's sexual inclination might already be decided before one is aware of its presence, the young adolescent has yet to make a determination. Adolescents are not yet sexual—heterosexual, homosexual, or otherwise. The attainment of adult sexuality is a slow process and, regardless of the object of one's sexuality, lasting fulfillment lies in the attainment of true intimacy rather than mere sexual gratification.

The question of sexual orientation in one's offspring provokes much anxiety in parents. The world being what it is, the adolescent with a homosexual orientation faces many problems. Some homosexual adolescents become acutely depressed, and more than a few adolescent suicides originate in the fear of homosexuality or the social stresses attached to it. The social stresses can be overwhelming. However, like most of life's other stresses, social stresses can be endured if one is blessed with the love and understanding of one's family, for it is within the family that one can seek solace during periods of adversity.

Early Adolescent Sexual Activity

Sexual behavior can bring pleasurable feelings in and of itself. It is one of the many ways human beings relate to one another. There are positive implications of the sexual act over and above the physical release. There are symbolic meanings attached to the act that tend to validate one's attractiveness and worthiness.

The risks of sexual activity in the early adolescent are significant. And adolescents receive conflicting messages from many sources about whether they should have sex: the popular media, schools, friends, adults, and even parents.

Popular Media Encourages Sex

Certainly there are many outside sources that communicate the meaning of being a man or woman to the emerging adolescent, such as books, movies, and television, and even friend's parents.

In wondering how to become a man, the young adolescent male asks himself, "What are the things that men do, which when done by me will make me a man?" He surveys a wide range of activities and quickly learns that one of the things that men do is have sex with women. In his pre-Aristotelian type of logic, he concludes that having sex with a woman means he will be a man. Or a 13-year-old girl may conclude that womanhood means "going all the way" with a male.

And why should parents be surprised at such logic? Everything around adolescents fairly shrieks of the sexual component of genderhood. Sexual activity is promoted as the be all and end all. Sex sells toothpaste. Adolescents are urged to be alluring, attractive, and popular. Wherever adolescents turn, they see adulthood represented as sexual success.

Well, it's true! Sexual intercourse is one of the things men and women do together—but it is only one of the ways they relate. Perhaps it is the easiest part of being an adult; certainly, it is one of the most pleasant. It requires little in the way of instruction or practice. Most healthy adults possess a strong drive for sexual gratification. The future of the race depends on it. It is an essential aspect of a well-adjusted and healthy adulthood.

Parents Can Give Mixed Messages Regarding Sex

It is not true that all adolescents are going to "do it" anyway. Many of them draw strength from the knowledge that their parents would be disappointed if they got themselves into trouble. These are the adolescents whose parents have been successful in passing on their values and in developing the sort of relationship with their children that will give them good cause for shaping their lives by the same values. The danger is not that parents will somehow fail to keep their children safe, but that somehow or other they will confuse them about their values or about their expectations for their behavior.

Remember that communication with children consists of not only the content of the spoken words, but also the process of the communication, which at times can belie the meaning of the spoken words. For example, some parents believe that they should put their daughter on contraceptive pills "just in case." They say, "If we did not put her on the pill and she happened to get pregnant, it would be our fault." I disagree on two premises. First, no one "happens" to get pregnant; deciding to have sex is a very deliberate act. Second, it would not be the parents' fault. Parents have the duty to talk with their children about the dangers of the world, but they can't prevent the dangers. They can only let them know about the physical and psychological risks of their behavior. True, adolescents must eventually take control of their own lives. But it is best to counsel them about getting their heads on straight before asking them to begin making decisions regarding behavior that carries risks.

The only way in which these parents might be at fault is by giving their daughter a mixed message. Although they tell her not to have sex, their message is undercut by their providing the birth control pills, which in essence says, "Go ahead and have sex." It would be similar to telling your children, "Don't smoke, but here is a carton of filter tipped, low-tar cigarettes just in case you decide to experiment." Parents must think about the implications hidden in the discussions around the use of birth control pills or devices. Telling an adolescent boy, "Be sure to take your condoms, son" leaves little doubt as to parental expectations for the outcome of their son's date.

Dangers of Early
Adolescent Sexual Activity

Early adolescent sexual activity carries with it a number of jeopardies, some of which are not all that apparent—certainly not to the adolescent, but sometimes not even to parents or other adults. Some of the more obvious dangers are teenage pregnancies and venereal disease. As a psychiatrist, I am concerned about the psychological risks. There is no condom or antibiotic that will provide psychological protection. I think adolescents need to abstain from sexual intercourse until they have reached a degree of psychological maturity at least to the extent that the major struggles of adolescence have been resolved.

Sexually Transmitted Diseases

One must be wary of proposing simple solutions to common problems—and beware of the message being sent to adolescents. In distributing birth control pills, one implicit message being sent regarding the dangers of early adolescent sexual activity is "Just

don't get pregnant!" Is that the only danger? Although birth control pills can prevent pregnancy if used in a proper and responsible
way, they won't prevent AIDS, gonorrhea, or syphilis.

Alternatively, if every adolescent boy could be provided with a
lifetime supply of condoms, would that prevent venereal disease?
Perhaps, if they were used properly and responsibly. But how can
you ensure that an adolescent boy uses condoms "properly and responsibly?" How do you get him to be proper and responsible
about cleaning up his room? Or about schoolwork? Or his driving?
Not easily!

Teenage Pregnancies

Very few adolescent girls want to get pregnant. Most of those who
do get pregnant were looking for something else in their sexual relationship. Some want to be needed by and feel close to another human being. So great is the need for acceptance, the vulnerable
adolescent exposes herself to risk. For that lonely and vulnerable girl,
at some level, the risk is not that of becoming pregnant. The risk is
being unimportant! The risk is losing what she has with that special
person at that moment. At that moment she matters to someone.

Experience has shown that teenage pregnancies will not be
eliminated simply by distributing birth control pills to adolescent
girls who are likely to give birth to an illegitimate child. Again, the
problem is in the message that is being given to these adolescents:
"Have sex, *safely!*" What the young adolescent hears is, "*Have sex,*
safely." It is not the strategy of providing education about birth
control that is flawed, but the premise upon which that strategy is
founded: Adolescents are going to have sex anyway, so let's simply
make certain that they perform in a proper and responsible manner.
Unwittingly, adults are contributing to the problem, even as they
try to solve it.

When an adolescent girl becomes pregnant, parents need to see
the event as a major challenge to their parental wisdom. Like other
crises of parenthood, this also offers opportunity as well as much
anxiety. Most parents are prepared to stand by their child no matter
what happens, and most have, at one time or another, so declared.
Here, then, is the challenge. I have known many young female ado-

lescents who have become pregnant and who have participated in the painful deliberations that followed between them and their parents. Although there were no easy solutions, many of these adolescents and parents later saw the event as one which drew them closer together.

When a young adolescent girl discovers that she is pregnant, her first thought is, "My mother will kill me." Her second thought is, "My father will kill my boyfriend." Seldom does either event occur. Do parents get upset? You bet! Most of the pregnant young adolescents I have known were terrified at the prospect of telling their parents. Most of them told their mother first and then their mother told their father. Think about how frightening it would be at age 13 to be pregnant and to know that you have to tell your parents. Some girls just can't face that and, instead, try to terminate the pregnancy or to terminate themselves.

I doubt there is a parent anywhere who has not thought about this. Parents must ask themselves, "Would our daughter have the courage to come and tell us if she were pregnant?" It might take a lot of courage for your daughter to face you. What would that be like, having to face you? Whether your child is willing to bring you this bad news will greatly depend upon what your response has been to other unpleasant news. It will help if parents have earned a reputation with their children over the years based on many things, not the least of which is their capacity for listening in order to understand.

Psychological Impact of Early Adolescent Sexual Activity

What worries me most about early adolescent sexual intercourse is the psychological impact it has on the participants. Herein can lie a wound far more grievous than meets the eye. It lies buried in the emerging gender identity. There are consequences for both the male and the female. Each is learning about the opposite gender and being taught by each other. What does each learn?

Impact on males. There is nothing more urgent than a 13-year-old boy drenched in testosterone and seeking release from his sexual tension. He is prepared to do or say almost anything as he negotiates an agreement that will bring him release. He'll even say, "I love you!" At a time when he should be learning how to become responsible for himself and eventually responsible for another, he finds himself seeking and finding immediate gratification. While learning what it means to be a man, the sexually active young adolescent male learns that the female is supposed to see to it that nothing happens, and that if she gets pregnant, she will take care of it. He learns that men aren't supposed to concern themselves about things like that. That young adolescent male not only learns something about manhood that will lead to an erosion of his value as a caregiver and the provider of security, but he develops an arrogant and insufferable attitude about women—and a distorted view of what it means to be a man.

One of the hallmarks of psychological maturity is the capacity to postpone immediate gratification for future reward. The impulsive, immature adolescent male has difficulty in imposing restraints of any sort upon himself. Restraints on his anger and physical combativeness are aided by the sanctions that society imposes upon him. Retaliation by others can also be educational in that process. But when society removes sanctions against aggressive violence, the adolescent male might find it more difficult to impose limits upon himself. The same applies to sexual activity. When society (or parents) remove sanctions against adolescent sexual activity, it makes abstaining more difficult.

Impact on females.   Between ages 13 and 20, a female adolescent will learn what it means to be a woman. By her early teenage years, she has already begun elaborating a sense of gender identity and will weave the fabric of that identity using what she is taught, what she will learn from the significant people in her life, and the experiences she encounters along the way. Much of that will be influenced by knowledge she already possesses, as well as how she will come to feel about herself as a woman and as an individual. Later, she will learn what men are like, but first she must come to know what women are like.

A young female may meet a young male who, yearning for sexual release, will do or say anything to gain that release. This teaches the female adolescent that men are only interested in sex and that that is what women are for! She learns that having sex with males pleases them. In her adolescent thought processes, she concludes that one of the things a woman is supposed to do is please men. She also learns that, if she is willing to have sex with a man, she can get almost anything she wants! The central theme of her sexual education at this critically important time in her psychological life is that women are here to take care of men. She learns that males are the important gender. She learns a terrible lesson that females are less important. The young female who has "decided to become sexually active" just as she is formulating a concept of womanhood is rendered a terrible disservice.

One of the very valuable sources of information about femaleness will be her girlfriends. Girlfriends help her contemplate femaleness by offering her close companions who see the world through similar eyes. But when an adolescent girl becomes sexually active, she spends more and more time with a male and less and less time with females as she begins to discount women. Not only is she getting a distorted view of herself as a woman, but she also loses the opportunity to learn of the joy that comes from a close companionship with another woman.

Once sexual behavior is put into motion, it develops an almost irresistible momentum. How to have sex is not all that difficult to learn and needs little in the way of practice. On the other hand, how to be a woman, in the broadest sense of the word, is a slow process. Early adolescent sexual activity shifts the emphasis from the broad context of womanhood and directs it toward the mastering of sexual techniques and sexual gratification.

It is possible to prevent both teenage pregnancies and sexually transmitted diseases. But it is not so easy to rework one's gender identity once it has been developed. This, then, is that grievous wound that is hidden from view and buried in an immature concept of self—a wound immune to all known antibiotics.

Maturity Enhances Sexuality

Many things contribute to one's sense of gender integrity. Not all of the malformations can be laid at the door of early adolescent sexual activity. Other influences in an adolescent's life might have deleterious consequences. But, regardless of what has occurred before in an adolescent's life, this struggle to evolve a healthy concept of self needs time.

A 21-year-old individual who becomes sexually active does so on a firmer ego structure than does a 13-year-old. Not only is the young adult more able to manage the unplanned consequences of his or her behavior, but he or she will have done the necessary psychological work and be less psychologically vulnerable to any unpleasant consequences. If adolescents postpone becoming sexually active until they reach early adulthood, they will have a greater chance for a satisfactory and fulfilling relationship with another human being.

Sexuality, Adolescents, and Families

Forcing an Adolescent to Abstain From Sex

How do parents see to it that their adolescent abstains from sexual intercourse? The answer is that they can't, and they shouldn't try. It is quite difficult to enforce abstention. Moreover, parental efforts to enforce abstention can become counterproductive as they set up control issues that adolescents feel they must oppose. Moreover, those efforts unintentionally imply that it is indeed the parents' responsibility to provide sexual safety for their adolescent. The frightening part for parents is that there is no sexual safety short of abstention, and abstention is in the hands of a not yet psychologically mature adolescent.

Parents must remain alert to the fact that adolescents are especially given to reading into parental messages interpretations never dreamed of by their parents. "Don't take the car to McDonalds" becomes "But it's okay to hang out at Burger King!" "Don't let me catch you speeding" can come to mean "Don't let me know about it." Communication with the adolescent is never simple or unadorned. There are always explicit and implicit messages in what seem to be simple communications. This is especially so when the communication is one with highly charged emotional components.

So what can parents do? They can ensure that they have a good relationship with their adolescent, the kind of relationship that will make him or her want to go to his or her parents and talk, especially about the things that are hard for him or her to tell us. (See also Chapter 3 on communication with adolescents.) I think adolescents need parental support and encouragement to understand the challenges of adolescent psychological growth—the scary parts as well as the wonderful parts.

Sex education in school can be helpful, but I am not convinced that it can't or shouldn't be done at home. It would be helpful if those who teach sex education in the schools were of such a level of maturity that they understand not only the mechanics of sexual intercourse but also possess an acute sense of responsibility for the many other ways humans relate to one another. Teaching this is a task for a mature, stable, emotionally sound individual. It should not be handed over to either Penelope Prude or Susie Swinger.

Parents and Their Children's Sexuality

Adolescents worry about the unfolding of their sexuality but not as much as their parents do. Something happens to adults when their offspring become capable of reproducing. Initially, parents tend to deny the sexuality of their adolescent, not unlike how adolescents tend to deny the sexuality of their parents. But as each day into adolescence passes, parents are compelled to recognize these changes.

An adolescent's emerging sexuality makes a subtle, but disturbing, declaration about the parents and where they are in their own life cycle. A parent might think, if she is old enough to conceive, then I am old enough to be a grandparent!

But these changes do more than redefine parents. A major increase in the parental sense of responsibility ensues. What has been a responsibility for the general well-being of their child now becomes more specific, as well as broader. Not only are parents now bound to keep harm away from their child but also to keep their child away from harm. Young adults believe that their parents somehow try to dictate to them about their sex life and sexual freedom and that it is none of their parents' business. Even in the earlier years of being a parent, adults tend to identify with those who are struggling against the yoke of parental authority. But attitudes change slowly, especially when one becomes the parent of an adolescent. Parents who only a few short years ago allied themselves with those who were being subjected to unwarranted controls by the older generation suddenly find themselves the parents of young adults and, hence, have become part of the "older generation." It is in this role that parents begin to urge their adolescents to move toward a more responsible application of sexual restraint, just as their parents did before them.

A Strong Marital Relationship Inhibits Incest

Intact families endure stressful events, such as an adolescent's increasing sexuality, better when the parents have a strong parental and marital relationship. Incest is not likely to occur when a fulfilling marital relationship exists between parents, step or otherwise. The blossoming of gender fulfillment in one's children brings more than anxiety. Suddenly, standing there before a father is the embodiment of the 17-year-old girl he fell in love with so many years ago. How can he help but feel nostalgia and tenderness? A mother looks at her adolescent son and can see his father as he used to be. Cherished memories flood adults when their children begin to experience the excitement of their emerging sexuality. It is not necessarily a problem, but it is a challenge.

Changes in Relationships With Parents

Once adolescents move into increased sexuality, their relationship with their parents can become suddenly tumultuous without the parents or adolescents understanding what is happening or why. A 37-year-old mother of three children sat in my office and wept as she recounted repeated battles with her 13-year-old son.

> He disagrees with everything I say. I feel overwhelmed by the repeated battles. Nothing I do or say pleases him anymore. He

gets along well with his father, but sometimes I think he hates me. And the frustrating part is that he has always been a good boy. We have always been close and affectionate. But now he just doesn't even like me anymore.

Perhaps you have already sensed what was happening. It was apparent to me that not only was this parent becoming less needed, but that this young adolescent male in fact did not hate his mother. On the contrary, he loved his mother very much. And that terrified him! He found himself involved in a warm, close, and loving relationship with an attractive female with whom he lived in intimate closeness. Adolescents tend to equate love with sex. I'm not suggesting that either mother or son had any conscious sexual feelings for each other. The relationship was a good one. It was a close relationship—too close for comfort. The only way the son was able to put some distance between himself and his mother was by keeping her at arms' length in repeated battles.

When this mother came to understand that her son's fault finding and fighting with her were defensive maneuvers unconsciously employed to relieve vaguely defined fears, she felt better about herself and was able to give him some breathing room. Here was a mother who felt that she was not a good mother who was not trying hard enough. In reality, she was a very good mother who was doing too much.

The advent of impending adolescent sexuality within the family can have a somewhat disruptive effect for fathers also. All of a sudden, Daddy's little girl doesn't want to sit on his lap anymore. Not only that, she finds fault with him and avoids him. He's hurt. Another scenario might be that a father, accustomed to giving his daughter a big hug and a good-night kiss, discovers that his little girl has suddenly gotten all soft in the chest and he recoils from this nightly tradition. The girl doesn't understand why her father seems to avoid her lately.

Adolescents and New Stepfamilies

When an adolescent going through the turmoil of arriving sexuality becomes part of a new stepfamily, that reconstituted family can expect to deal with the same dynamics noted above in addition to some further complications. For example, a father who remarries and expects his 17-year-old son to treat his new sister as if she really were a sister expects a bit much. In an intact family, brothers and sisters have the comfort of developing appropriate taboos over years to protect themselves. In a reconstituted family, learning to live with a new parent, new child, or new sibling requires work, understanding, and effective communication in order to manage even the nonsexual aspects. Managing the sexual aspects requires all of the above and even more. Expecting adolescent children to immediately desexualize a new and attractive parent or sibling of the opposite gender is naive.

Conclusion

Emerging sexuality is part of the development of gender identity. But there is more to being a man than learning how to have sexual intercourse. More urgent is the need to develop a capacity for work, protection, loyalty, forbearance, compassion, and strength. A young adolescent male's future role as a man, husband, and father will depend upon qualities of character much more than a capacity for sexual intercourse.

For the girl on her way to becoming a woman, her reproductive capacity will validate her femaleness, but as with her opposite gender, the kind of woman she becomes will rest upon the foundation of a wide array of personal qualities. A capacity for nurturing, tenderness, loyalty, understanding, and the giving and receiving of affection will give definition to her womanhood. There is so much more to being a woman than the mere capacity for sexual intercourse.

Learning how to have sex is not very complicated. There are more important qualities that children must seek and find in their parents. If parents have been able to communicate the love they feel for their children to them, they will be seen as attractive models. If parents make themselves available to their children, the children will, for the most part, try to grow up and be like their parents.

Section III

Problems in Adolescence

Chapter 8

Adolescents' Risk-Taking Behavior

*E*verywhere I turn, I read of outrageous adolescent behavior, interspersed with dire predictions of worse yet to come. It's enough to make parents want to hide their children or leave town with no forwarding address. Crime, drugs, sex, mental illness, and death—all seem to lurk in the path of the adolescent, whether the adolescent is the perpetrator or the one on the receiving end. More and more criminal acts carried out by younger and younger children seem to be the norm for the morning news. Ongoing drug abuse by adolescents is revealed in study after study. Suicide in young people has increased enormously during the past decade. Adolescent gangs roam the streets in our inner cities, asserting their "rights" on one another and the surrounding neighborhoods and neighbors. Teenage pregnancies, venereal diseases, rapes, and robberies are brought to us through the courtesy of our local adolescent.

Why Adolescents Take Risks

Some of the things adolescents do involve great risk to their general well-being, their health—both mental and physical, and their life. Adolescents are prone to risk. "Take a chance" is an attractive challenge to adolescents. Psychiatrists have no absolute explanation of why adolescents put themselves at risk. Some psychiatrists write about an innate death wish that resides in all people. They suggest that people enjoy having close calls. Some believe that there is an excitement to having a narrow miss. Most people would greatly appreciate being missed and would prefer that it not even come close to being a narrow miss.

In trying to understand why adolescents do some of the things that cause concern in adults, it helps to keep in mind the adolescent process and its implications.

Adolescents' Sense of Omnipotence

Some psychiatrists believe that adolescents' risk-taking behavior is grounded in what is called the *omnipotence of adolescence*. It is this sense of omnipotence that leads adolescents to a belief in their own invulnerability. There does seem to be a sense of omnipotence in adolescents, and that belief undoubtedly fuels their risk-taking behavior. To adolescents, the world beckons. Anything is possible.

Where do they find this sense of omnipotence? Partially it comes from the emergence of newly found strength and newly found ability. A fully developed and fresh body offers a heady brew. It's true that adolescents can now do things for which they previously were not prepared. Adulthood looms just ahead.

The omnipotence of adolescence is more easily understood if one reminds oneself of the tasks the adolescent now performs. The sense of power in the adolescent represents a transfer of powerfulness from previously held concepts of parents. Adolescents now take back the power invested in their protectors so long ago. "They are no longer all powerful; I am no longer helpless" is an exciting discovery.

Adolescents' Desire to Move Into Adulthood

The adolescent faces the constant temptation of false shortcuts to adulthood offering instant gratification, such as the following:

◆ Little children are not allowed to smoke. Adults smoke; therefore, if I smoke, I am an adult.

◆ Little children must not use drugs. Adults use drugs; therefore, if I use drugs, I am an adult.

◆ Little children do not have sex. Adults have sex; therefore, if I have sex, I am an adult.

Driven by a longing for adult status, armed with a sense of invulnerability, and still lacking some of life's chastising experiences, the adolescent plunges ahead believing that misfortune will befall only other people. Unable to postpone immediate gratification for future reward, the emotionally immature adolescent throws caution to the wind. Such high-risk behavior can maladaptively lead to a fixation at an adolescent rather than adult level of development.

This shift of new power is accomplished by one who is, in some ways, not yet ready for it. Adolescents acquire enormous strength and attractiveness well before developing the wisdom for their judicious use. They have not yet had the experiences that will help them perceive the potential consequences for the misuse of these new abilities. Only slowly do they develop a sense of *consequentiality,* a fancy word that merely means an understanding of cause and effect. Slowly, we all must learn our way through life. And the length of that life bears a striking relationship with the risks we take and the wisdom we acquire for the management of those risks.

Constructive Risks Can Promote Growth

Risk taking can be a constructive part of adolescents' lives. Adolescents should be curious about themselves and the limits of their potential. Adults applaud the adolescent who takes constructive risks. For example, the adolescent who throws caution to the wind and strives to see how smart he or she is in achieving academic excellence is applauded.

Valuable lessons can be learned from taking risks. I recall a young man whose mother urged him not to climb the fence that surrounded his family's home. He assured his mother that he had no intention of falling and continued his climb. The broken collar bone that he received after falling from the fence tended toward the improvement of his climbing skills and served as an early introduction to the concept of cause and effect.

Without risk, new heights are never reached. There was a time when it was an accepted fact that no one could run a mile in less than 4 minutes. A young man named Roger Bannister believed that with training, he could break that barrier. He took a chance and prevailed. Parents want their adolescents to have faith in themselves and to apply themselves and succeed. One mother complained that her 10-year-old son took great delight in climbing a tree in his backyard as high as he could go. She was terrified that he would fall. She wasn't particularly impressed when I suggested that the view from the top can be so exhilarating that it might make the climb and the risk worth it all. I suggested that he might someday rise to other great heights. I gave her little consolation at the time. But today he is a very successful physician who graduated "at the top" of his class.

Adolescents and Destructive Risks

Constructive risks are easy to support and understand. It's more difficult to understand why adolescents take risks that can lead to destructive ends, such as taking drugs, drinking alcohol, and risking sexually transmitted diseases and teenage pregnancies; these demand our attention.

Adolescents Who Take Destructive Risks

Adolescents come with different strengths and liabilities that will determine the level of risk they are willing to take. Some adolescents will take great risks. Some will live dangerously and die young. Some won't die right away but will begin a process of risk taking that will eventually lead to death or disability. Some won't become physically disabled but will, as a consequence of risk-taking behavior, find themselves psychologically or economically disabled. For example, some adolescents will not experiment with drugs regardless of the temptation and peer pressure, some will experiment and decide against any further use, and still others will experiment and continue to use a particular drug but never become addicted. As another example, a female adolescent, yearning for love, acceptance, or just simply adulthood, might become sexually active and risk finding herself permanently dependent and economically disabled as she struggles to raise the child she had as a teenager. Or there is the adolescent who feels he or she has no control over his or her life and might attempt to take control through repeated risk taking, which eventually leads to conflict with the law.

Grossman et al. (1992) suggested that certain factors in the lives of adolescents help them in their adaptation: at least a minimal amount of self-esteem, a feeling that they have some control over their lives, a feeling that there is a sense of cohesion in their families, and the ability to communicate well with at least one of their parents. But even well-adjusted adolescents can do dumb things. "I dare you," can be the beginning of something foolish. Most foolish acts are nonfatal, just foolish.

The vulnerable ones are those who yearn for attention or acceptance. These children are the ones who will sometimes risk their life rather than repudiate the attention that comes from "I dare you!" These are the children who will be more likely to accept the overtures of an impassioned lover. Wanting desperately to hear "I love you" and wanting desperately to say "I love you," the lonely feel less alone if they can somehow matter to someone—maybe anyone!

Look Beyond Risk-Taking Behavior

As a psychiatrist, I am inclined to look not only at the behavior but also at the forces that shape that behavior. Some of the adolescent's behavior is so risky, it is difficult to look beyond it for an explanation. Drug abuse might reflect some form of disarray in the adolescent's life, but the symptom of that disarray is a most compelling one. In fact, it is so compelling that many parents and some treatment facilities focus only on the behavior while completely overlooking the cause of it. It is difficult to be philosophically curious about hidden causes while an adolescent's life seems to be going madly toward its ending. On the other hand, unless the cause of self-destructive behavior is sought, the behavior will occur again and again.

There is no single cause involved in adolescent self-destructive behavior. But there is almost always an underlying cause. And although risk-taking behavior embraces seemingly different kinds of behavior, there is a kinship of purpose in its use. In their worldwide study of adolescents, Offer et al. (1988) determined that 80% of all adolescents function in a healthy manner, whereas about 20% have some emotional disturbance, only one-fourth of whom receive adequate help. They emphasized that dysfunctional adolescents experience their disability during a critical period in their life when significant changes are taking place. Depression or lowered self-esteem that might otherwise be detected might simply be attributed to adolescent struggles. These symptoms might then go unnoticed into adulthood. Offer et al. urge clinicians to seek underlying causes.

Before understanding why a certain behavior is taking place, one needs to understand exactly what that behavior is. For example, knowing what substance is being consumed will help me understand what it does to the adolescent. But I also want to know what it does *for* the adolescent, which depends upon that adolescent's particular qualities—his or her needs and how well he or she is equipped to find adaptive methods in meeting those needs. In reviewing destructive behavior, one must keep in mind that it doesn't always involve abusing a substance. An adolescent might neither drink nor take drugs nor manifest any other colorful or compelling symptomatology, but might simply quietly experience some sort of malignant dysfunction that can lead to destruction.

The tragedy lies in the danger that can result from the symptomatology as well as the danger that is hidden behind the symptomatology! So compelling can symptomatology be, that it becomes tempting to combat it alone without seeking that which it hides, as might have occurred in the following example:

Mitzy, a 17-year-old girl, had used drugs since age 15. She had been treated twice for drug intoxication, both instances of which had been thought to be the result of accidental overdoses. Her father had died when she was age 10, and her mother remarried when Mitzy was age 12. The marriage was satisfactory but loveless. Mitzy disliked her stepfather but seldom complained.

During her treatment for drug abuse, Mitzy continued to use drugs. She was moody but mostly depressed. Both parents complained about Mitzy's drug problem and ascribed her poor grades and depression to her using drugs. Once we insisted that the family participate in family treatment, the parents' marital discord soon became apparent. Shortly thereafter, Mitzy admitted to using drugs for 2 years and to having sexual intercourse with her stepfather for 3 years. What had been diagnosed as a drug problem proved to be an incest problem. If we had focused all of our attention on Mitzy's drug problem, we could have missed a very pathological dysfunction hiding behind drug abuse.

Of course, Mitzy compounded her problem of incest by drug abuse. On the other hand, drug abuse became a way for her to manage her anger, fear, and guilt. She felt that she needed the drugs she used. What she really needed most of all was a resolution of the underlying pathological relationship with her stepfather.

Had we not looked beyond the drug abuse, we might have contented ourselves by seeing to it that Mitzy "stop using drugs." If our treatment had consisted only of educating her to the danger of drugs, we would have unwittingly colluded in the preservation of Mitzy's anguish and despair. Once treatment was focused on the dysfunctional relationship between Mitzy's mother and stepfather, and that was brought to resolution, Mitzy no longer needed and no longer used drugs.

This case demonstrates the importance a strong parental coalition has in children's lives. Mitzy's parents failed to meet the needs of each other, one result of which was that the stepfather reached across the generational boundary and involved himself in a need-fulfilling relationship with his stepdaughter. Although Mitzy indulged in risk-taking behavior by her use of drugs, it is clear that drug use was her maladaptive effort to solve a desperate matter.

The following case example is similar in that the dysfunctional behavior was hiding a deeper problem:

Sarah was brought to me when she was age 14. Her parents told me that she was an alcoholic. Indeed, Sarah agreed with their assessment and willingly described herself as an alcoholic. Sarah had actually begun drinking at age 13. Careful and extensive evaluation of Sarah and her family revealed seriously disturbed relationships within the family. At the time of Sarah's admission to the adolescent psychiatric ward, her father was psychotic and delusional. He was actively hallucinating but had become adept at hiding the evidence. Sarah's mother was malignantly depressed and suicidal. She knew something was wrong with her husband but had been unable to persuade him to get help. He was able to continue working but was morose, suspicious, and reclusive. Sarah's younger brother had begged her to "do something" to get help. Sarah had no idea how to "do something" and felt helpless. Then she discovered alcohol. She would drink at night to help her sleep. Sarah drank for almost a year before her parents realized that they needed to get help—for Sarah! Help for Sarah brought help for her father. Help for her father brought help for her mother. It took Sarah over a year to "do something." By doing more than seeing Sarah as an alcoholic, we were able to get at the underlying pathology and treat the cause of this family's dysfunction.

Adolescents jeopardize their lives in complex ways. The foregoing cases cover only a narrow band of risk-taking behavior.

Why Parents Have Trouble Understanding Adolescents' Risky Behavior

There is a wide range of behavior indulged in by adolescents that not only perplexes adults but also maims, disables, or kills adolescents. Not all of it leads to death. Some behavior leads to a lifelong disability. "Why do they do it?" I am asked. My temptation is to say, "Beats me" or "I haven't the foggiest idea!" But I can't. I must know.

Adults are at a disadvantage in trying to understand adolescent behavior, especially parents, because it is not easy to be objective about their children. This is because they are not objects; they're their children. They love them, worry about them, and are scared for them. How can parents think calmly, quietly, and dispassionately when fear clutches them?

One answer is to seek advice from someone who isn't deeply invested in or scared about their children. Many parents get advice from other parents. It's easier to think clearly when he or she is not your child. But, after all else has failed, some parents turn to mental health professionals. They meet with some success in finding answers. Why? Partly because they are able to be objective, and perhaps more importantly because they are willing to consider explanations that do not make sense.

There is something about adolescent behavior that defies logic. Almost invariably, parents try to apply adult logic to their understanding of the adolescent. In a sense, this wonderful capacity, so useful in the adult world, can be a hindrance in the adolescent's world. Illogical behavior cannot be understood using logical thought. But if one can put aside adult logic momentarily and consider explanations that are illogical, one might glean an explanation of why a particular adolescent is doing things that don't otherwise make sense. Things are not always the way they seem, as in the following example:

Chris had made very good grades throughout his school career. In the seventh grade, he did less well. His mother pressed him to do better. He did worse. Moving into a part of his life that would ordinarily give him some of the privileges of adulthood, he found himself subjected to a great deal of parental restrictions and directions. His mother brought Chris to me. "I can't understand it," she said. "He used to make good grades. Now I dread seeing his report card. I have put him on restriction again and again. He tells me that I nag him. I feel trapped. I guess I am on his back a lot. It sure would be easier for me if he would live up to his potential," she explained. I agreed to see Chris for a few visits in hopes of shedding some light on the situation.

Chris complained about his mother's "bugging" him about his grades. "I hate it. She makes me feel like a child. I wish she would stop," was his constant refrain when talking with me. I scratched my head. Here were two intelligent people caught in a situation that neither of them liked. And yet, it continued on and on. It didn't make sense. There was no logic in it.

But, in an illogical way the current situation made sense. The situation was unpleasant, maladaptive, and counterproductive, but were there benefits or advantages to this impasse? Maybe. I could easily see what all of this was doing to these two people. What was not as easily seen was what all of this was doing *for* these two people.

After hearing Chris complain about his mother's bugging him about his grades over and over, I said to him, "You know, Chris, I'm confused. You tell me that you don't like having your mother nag you about your grades, and yet you very carefully avoid doing the one thing that would guarantee getting her off your back." "What's that?," he asked. "Making good grades," I replied. I could see in his face a puzzled look as he processed the thought. It took him a minute to speak. "Hmmm, I do not know. I wonder why," he mused.

I responded, "I don't know, Chris. I can only guess. I know your mother loves you very much and wants you to grow up. But I guess she wants to keep on being important to you. As long as you make poor grades, you'll be a little boy in her eyes. One who very much needs his mother!" I theorized. Chris scowled at me. "That doesn't make sense!" he retorted. "Oh?" I asked. "So you feel that's not the case?" I asked. "Well, you may be right," I confessed and said no more.

I didn't see Chris for several weeks. Upon his return, he chatted on and on. Finally he said, "I've been thinking about what you said. You may be right." "Oh?" I asked. "Yeah, I think she's doing better since my grades have improved," he informed me. "Hmmm, that's very interesting!" I added.

Upon reflection, what had not originally made sense was now more understandable. There were forces at work between Chris and his mother that greatly influenced their struggle. Those forces were not all that apparent, but having some understanding of the great challenges that Chris encountered in his movement away from childhood helped me look for explanations that were not on the surface, and my refusal to demand that he agree with my analysis allowed him to come to the same conclusion after "thinking about it."

What Parents Can Do to Prevent Risky Behavior

Believe in Their Children

One way parents can prevent risky behavior is to believe in their children. Parents raise their children in the best manner they can,

trying to inculcate good values in them. After a child reaches adolescence, parents must learn to trust their child.

Sometimes parents are so afraid their adolescents will get into
trouble that they begin to do the sort of things that will foster an
adversarial relationship with their children, all in the guise of helping, as in the following case example:

> Dottie was a 16-year-old girl whose parents were afraid she would
> get into trouble. She hadn't. But they asked: "Would you be will-
> ing to talk with her and warn her about drugs?"
>
> What I saw was an attractive and effervescent adolescent
> who was popular with others, productive in her schoolwork, and
> the recipient of much parental love and protection. Dottie told
> me, "I play basketball on my high school team. I love it. It's fun.
> When we win, I get real excited. I have to wait until I calm down
> before going home or Mom will think I'm high on some kind of
> drug. She gets up real close looking at my pupils to see if they are
> dilated and to smell my breath to see if I've been drinking. I don't
> do either. I wish my parents would trust me more. Would you be
> willing to talk with them for me?"

Help Adolescents Not Need to Engage in Risky Behavior

What can parents do to somehow help their adolescents face these
risky times? The answer is that parents cannot prevent the destructive behavior, but they can help adolescents not need to engage in
such behavior. Parents can do this by providing a loving, caring environment that will encourage an adolescent to seek autonomy and
independence at the right pace. Guidelines for accomplishing this
include the following:

1. *Do not wait until something goes wrong.* Develop the kind of relationship with your child that will foster open communication
   and mutual trust. Encourage his or her clumsy efforts to talk
   with you about his or her feelings—fear, anger, and sadness.
   Learn how to "show and tell" your love for your child, as well
   as your admiration for the kind of person he or she is becoming.

2. *Accept that you are going to make mistakes and manage them well.*
By the time children reach adolescence, parents will have had a
wealth of opportunities for mistakes. How they manage those
mistakes will have a bearing on their parenthood and how they
feel about themselves as individuals and as parents. How they
manage those mistakes will also set a pattern of response for
their children as they attempt to manage their own mistakes—
all of which goes straight to the heart of accepting the responsibility for one's behavior.

3. *Model for your children the living wisdom of personal responsibility.*
Be circumspect in how you conduct your life.

Parents conduct a demonstration project that conveys to
their children how to care for another human being. It is an
experiment in living conducted in the laboratory of the home.
Because it is not possible to be a child's permanent shield
against danger, parents should help their child learn how to accept responsibility for his or her actions.

It is human to want to relieve any feelings of anxiety or guilt.
When the consequences of behavior are not what one wishes,
one might seek an explanation outside of himself or herself in
order to provide relief from the bad feelings that are engendered
by the behavior. Externalizing blame to others or to circumstances beyond one's control tends to relieve guilt. But the price
paid for that relief is a feeling of helplessness and a loss of control of one's life. "It was their fault" or "I couldn't help it" suggests that others are in charge of one's life. Children who see
their parents doing this will probably follow suit. On the other
hand, when children see their parents searching for answers
inside themselves, they will learn to follow that behavior.

4. *Teach children that out of self-responsibility comes self-discipline; out
of self-discipline comes self-respect.* As children are able to accept
the responsibility for the things in their lives that do not go
well, so they will begin to give themselves credit for those
things that do go well. It is the ability to impose responsibility
for their lives upon themselves that will lead children to
self-responsibility. It is this self-responsibility that brings them
to self-discipline. From this ability to impose discipline upon
themselves, children will come to know self-respect. Adoles-

cents who are able to feel genuine respect for themselves are in a much stronger position to safeguard not only themselves but also those for whom they become responsible.

5. *Emphasize that each person is in charge of only himself or herself.* Individuals who can reflect on their actions with a degree of compassion and understanding of why things went wrong and what their role was in the process can tap into a source of enormous power. They discover that for better or worse their destiny is in their own hands. They determine that they alone can make their life better.

Conclusion

Life is a continuing risk. At any moment, risk can destroy life or seriously compromise it. But there is also the risk of a successful and full life lived in productive harmony with the environment and with fellow humans. Learning to accept responsibility for the management of our lives will help us in our assessment of the risks and opportunities that present themselves to us.

Parents want to protect children from dangerous risk. Up to a point, they can and they do. But each of us—including our children—must assume the ultimate responsibility for our own life and how it evolves. Because most of our wounds are self-inflicted, we must look inside ourselves for their healing and prevention. As we accept the responsibility for our fate—for better or for worse—we become more circumspect in how we conduct our lives. By modeling, we teach our children self-responsibility, self-discipline, and self-respect. Armed with these powerful shields, our children might be able to protect themselves.

Chapter 9

Serious Problems That Occur in Adolescence

*S*ometimes, no matter how hard you've tried, things go wrong! Although only a small number of adolescents experience serious psychiatric disorder to the extent of needing hospitalization, a larger number will require some form of help, or at least would benefit from it. How do parents know that their child needs that help? And how does one find the proper help?

Why Problems Develop

The earliest lesson I learned in working with adolescents was that, although some adolescents need the structured environment of a hospital to repair, the proper locale for this process is the bosom of their families. Only in understanding the context in which a child becomes disabled can one hope to bring about repair. Thus, when adolescents present to me with problems, I look at their home life to set their troubles in context.

Parents Try to Do Their Best

In my practice, I often came face to face with families that were in the midst of chaos. However, I can say that all these families were doing the best they could at the time. I never saw parents who were trying to create problems for their children. Instead, they were trying hard to do what was right—or what they thought was right. Some were confident that all of the problems in the family would disappear if the adolescent would straighten up and fly right, saying to me, "He's the problem, Doctor. If it weren't for him, we wouldn't be here. All we want him to do is cut his hair, come home on time, and do what we tell him to do. If you can make him behave, everything will be alright!" Such were the remarks of many of the parents who took part in our treatment program. Others came and brought a different view: "I feel terrible about my daughter's being here. It's all my fault. My wife says I'm too hard on the children. Maybe that's because she's too easy on them. I guess I'm the one who ought to be here!"

Problems Develop Gradually

Although I've had many adolescents come for care, none came for preventive care; that is, all were emergencies. But, in point of fact, none of them were real emergencies in the sense that they had just begun. Parents would describe painful events immediately preceding their decision to seek help, but upon reflection would recall that the problem had begun weeks, months, or even years earlier.

The usual scenario was that the parents would struggle with their child's difficulties over time, trying everything they knew to solve them. Then some event would precipitate their decision to go outside the family and seek help: a stolen automobile, a fist fight—sometimes between father and son, a pregnancy, an expulsion from school, an attempt to run away, the discovery of drugs or alcohol among the adolescent's possessions, or a suicidal or homicidal act—either attempted or completed. But more frequently, the events were not outrageous. Often they were simply "last straws."

As the scenario continued, almost invariably, one parent would try to convince the other that something was wrong. Or, frequently, fingers were pointed: husbands at wives, wives at husbands, parents at children, children at parents. So many of these families were terribly unhappy but struggled to keep their pain to themselves. There was little or no fun in their lives. Although the family members communicated with one another, they really never understood one another. They seemed to lack the skills needed to resolve conflicts within the family and felt that things were getting worse rather than better.

Problems Often Occur When Parents Are Unhappy Together

Even when parents are kind, considerate, and loving toward their children, things can go wrong. The problem can be tied to the parental relationship, as in the following example:

> Mattie, age 16, was an energetic and highly intelligent girl when I first saw her. I admitted her to the hospital following a suicide attempt. She had had three previous hospitalizations and had undergone psychiatric treatment for 3 years. She averaged about 10 months with each psychiatrist and then would find one reason or another to terminate treatment. Her parents were wealthy, socially prominent, and very loving toward Mattie, but not toward each other. They had reached a decision to seek divorce just before Mattie's first sign of psychiatric problems and her first hospitalization. Horrified that they might have contributed to Mattie's problems, her parents reconciled and worked toward saving the marriage. At that point, Mattie's condition improved.
>
> When the marriage began going downhill again, Mattie's illness returned, and she was admitted to another hospital. Another prolonged recovery for Mattie prompted her parents to try again to salvage their marriage. By the time I saw Mattie, she had begun questioning her role in her parents' marriage. Around age 16, she concluded that she could not be responsible for her parents' marriage. "I think I'll stop being sick. They get along much better when I'm sick. But I don't!" Her parents then resolved enough of their marital problems to stay together without any further "help" from Mattie.

Divorce and Adolescence

I have had the painful task of participating in legal hearings concerning the custody of children of divorce. I have never taken part in a custody hearing for children whose parents have cared for each other. Adolescence can be an especially bad time for a child to experience the divorce of his or her parents.

For the reasons I discuss throughout this book, adolescence is a particularly challenging and difficult time. First, as adolescents begin to redefine their view of their parents, they surrender some of the protection they have felt their parents provided. Second, they are attempting to elaborate a sense of who they are and how worthy they are of receiving others' love. This self-inquiry can lead to self-doubts. Third, as adolescents attempt to take on the characteristics of their gender, it is helpful to have a degree of harmony and participation with parents who provide the role model for them.

The occurrence of divorce makes these tasks more complicated but not impossible. Divorce can be corrosively destructive unless each parent can somehow come to terms with the anger that it engenders. For here lies the final wounding of children who become enmeshed in the bitterness of their parents' anger. I have seen the effects of divorce on children and adolescents. The adolescent adapts better to the dislocation of a parent and has a clearer understanding of the dynamics of the underlying problem than does the younger child.

Each age group has its own response to divorce. The adolescent is usually less frightened by parental separation but finds the loss of the same gender parent more problematic. All children secretly believe and even clearly state that their bad behavior has caused the divorce, but the adolescent perhaps less so. With the current high incidence of divorce, the adolescent has one or two friends who are equipped and ready to offer counsel.

It is true that divorce can be damaging to all children involved, but is it the act itself that does the damage? A group therapy session that I was conducting some years ago provided me with an interesting finding. One of the adolescents began talking about his parents' divorce, and it struck me that several other adolescents in the group were living in families that did not contain both biological parents. As I surveyed the group, I discovered that 9 of the 10 were living in homes minus at least one biological parent. I was struck by the fact that 9 of these 10 dysfunctional children were in so-called broken homes. Only 1 child was living with both biological parents. But the irony was that that child was the sickest of all of the 10 adolescents. He had severe schizophrenia, whereas the others all had problems but were not mentally ill.

Root of Problems
Could Be a Psychiatric Disorder

Some adolescents demonstrate problems that are serious enough to bring them to a psychiatrist. Some of these young people are desperately ill. Some attempt to kill themselves, sometimes making repeated attempts. Some of the suicide attempts are the result of major psychiatric disorders such as manic-depressive disorder or a schizophrenic disorder. Some come as a consequence of the commands of delusional or hallucinatory processes.

How can parents detect a psychiatric disorder in their child? It's not always easy because adolescents have different personalities, styles, and habits. And because of the conflicts they are encountering during this period of their life, their behavior can be quite erratic. Some of the behaviors noted below could be mistakenly interpreted as signs of a psychiatric disorder:

✦ Adolescents are ordinarily given to moodiness.
✦ Adolescents retreat to their rooms for hours at a time.
✦ Adolescents are irritable at times.
✦ Adolescents have appetites that can vary from picky to packing it in.
✦ Adolescents can get into patterns of sleeping late or waking early.

It is an overwhelming responsibility to be ever on alert, constantly ready to diagnose the earliest of psychiatric symptoms. Parents who maintain a constant watch over their children in anticipation that something might go wrong will leave little time for themselves. Moreover, it sets up a relationship that suggests their child doesn't have to be responsible for his or her life, that the parents will do it instead.

Major psychiatric disorders are more easily managed if their presence is announced with a flourish of abnormal behavior. But it doesn't always work that way. Schizophrenia can have a very quiet beginning. It can develop in a child who is by nature quiet and shy. Gradual withdrawal from social connections can be the only presenting symptom of such an illness. In a child who has been rambunctious, energetic, and outgoing, social withdrawal is more likely noted. But the quiet and inwardly turned child who begins to withdraw can do so almost unnoticed.

But most of the adolescents I saw were not seriously suicidal or burdened by severe mental illness. Most came from families who were bewildered and scared. Most were helped and returned to their home and families.

Once an adolescent's symptoms have been recognized as belonging to a particular psychiatric disorder, I am still cautious about placing a diagnosis on the condition, in part, because the adolescents are so incomplete but also because diagnoses have a way of becoming an imposed tyranny. Even more so, there lurks the danger that those diagnoses will become part of the warp and the woof of that fabric. I am a "schizophrenic" or an "alcoholic" or a "drug addict" or a "delinquent" becomes a way of viewing oneself in perpetuity. An adolescent's problems need to be understood for what they are, but one needs to recognize that lifelong concepts of self are being laid down at this time and have far-reaching implications for how a human being will come to feel about himself or herself.

Take Action Before
Problems Become Serious

How can parents know when something is wrong? They can't always. But there are a few strategies for ensuring the best outcome to any potential problems.

Periodically inquire how your adolescent's life is going. Parents can ask their adolescent the kind of questions about his or her life that will convey a sense of caring curiosity about the progress the adolescent feels he or she is making. Parental interest ought not wait until something is wrong. The following are examples of questions that probably would be perceived as not being nosy but simply as reflecting a genuine interest in the adolescent's life:

+ How are things going for you?
+ How are things at school and with your friends?
+ Did you settle things with your father?
+ How do you feel about the way you handled that?
+ What are your plans for the upcoming school year?

These questions not only gather information, but they also disseminate it in that during these kind of interactions parents tell their children that they are concerned about their life and what they are making of it. It tells them that their parents respect their ability to manage more and more of their life. These are "how" questions rather than "why" questions. "How" questions are more fun to hear. They seek opinions rather than justifications. Moreover, they make the process of talking with Mom or Dad something to look forward to rather than dread. Don't wait until something has gone wrong to begin talking with your adolescent.

Create an atmosphere in which your adolescent will want to tell you when something isn't right. It is important for parents to "have something going" with their children that will enhance the likelihood of the latter not waiting until something has gone wrong before talking with their parents. Such a relationship will make it not only easier for them to talk about what has gone wrong, but also will help in keeping things from going wrong in the first place. A relationship blessed by parents who understand what the adolescent process is about and who are sympathetic to their child's efforts to become an adult is one that fosters healthy growth for their adolescent and for themselves.

When something has gone wrong, you want your child to not be afraid to talk with you. And then, you must listen—listen in order to understand. Remain silent until your child has finished giving you the bad news. Then ask if there is anything else he or she wants to say. If he or she indicates that is all, check and see if you have understood correctly. "Let me see if I understand what you have told me. If I understand you correctly, X has happened, and you have done Y. Is that about right?" If it isn't, your son or daughter will tell you. Then it helps to let your child know that you are concerned about what has happened. To ask, "How do you plan to handle that?" lets him or her be responsible. When you ask, "What can I do to help?" you will be surprised at the number of times he or she will say, "You have already helped. You listened!"

Be a good consultant.   Your position as a parent should be that of a valued adult in the life of your child. By the time young people reach adolescence, they know right from wrong. They will have the fundamental equipment to take over the management of their lives but will still need a good consultant. That's you! And you have learned a thing or two during your life so far. The trouble is that parents can be impatient and overanxious. Parents want to make certain that problems turn out right—immediately!

A caring parent's attitude could be one of "I've gone through this before. I can save you a lot of trouble if you just do what I tell you to do," but there are several things wrong with this approach even though it is "good advice."

1. As much as adolescents want to become adults and do the adultlike thing, they want even more to stop being children. Sometimes the consultant's "good advice" sounds more like a commandment and seems to demand that the adolescent become a mirror image of the parent. In order to prove to themselves that they are no longer children, adolescents will find ways of thwarting parents' commandments.
2. "Good advice" often fails to recognize that there might be more than one way to solve a problem.
3. "Good advice" may not always be good—it may not always work.

A valuable "consultant" might handle a problem like this:

Son: Dad, I have a problem, and I need to talk with you about it.
Father: Sure, Jack, let's hear it.
Son: Well, it's about [fill in the blanks], and I am not sure how to handle it.

Father: Hmmm, I see. What have you tried so far?

  Son: Well, I have tried [fill in the blanks], but it didn't work.

Father: Have you thought about [fill in the blanks]?

  Son: Yes, and that didn't work either.

Father: Gosh, Jack, I don't know. I had a similar problem when I was your age, and I tried [fill in the blanks], and it didn't work for me either. And then I tried [fill in the blanks], and that seemed to help. I don't know if that would work in this case, but think about it.

Of course your words would be more appropriate in your own situation, but this might give you a starting point.

Recognize the importance of your adolescent's problem. In general, adolescents value their parents' opinions and will be greatly influenced by them. They realize that parents have had years of living experience. Part of the problem is that adolescents have difficulty in asking for advice or help. To do so admits to helplessness or ineptness. Part of the problem for parents is a tendency to discount the importance of the problem to their child. What appears trivial to adults can seem of great importance to adolescents.

Avoid a "know-it-all" attitude. Parents sometimes have the tendency to treat their advice as "gospel": "This is the way it ought to be done" or "This is what works" or "This is best." Even though parents know a lot, they seldom feel that they know it all. "My parents think they are perfect!" is a statement made by many adolescents. Again, the truth is that parents feel very imperfect. If there is one surefire antidote for parental feelings of perfection, it is having an adolescent child!

Let your adolescent develop his or her own judgment. Decision making is a task to be mastered through constant practice. Good judgment comes from carefully weighing the pros and cons of any issue. If adolescents are to become competent in this area, they must begin practicing the process at an early age. Once they reach adolescence, young people develop new mental skills and are able to analyze more complex situations, whereas adults have been making decisions for a long time and can make them quickly because of their vast experience. To really help your adolescent, help him or her learn the decision-making process rather than simply giving him or her the answer.

The advantages to giving answers to adolescents are that

✦ The problem is solved quickly.
✦ It impresses them with how much their parents know.
✦ It makes them look to their parents for future answers.
✦ It makes parents feel good and needed.

The advantages to helping adolescents *find* the answer are that

✦ It strengthens the parent-child relationship.
✦ It helps adolescents grow.
✦ It helps parents grow.

Recognize when help is wanted.   When something seems to be going wrong, parental interest should be reaffirmed and offers of help put forward. However, the help should be made available on the condition that the recipient wants it and that the helper is willing and able. Being willing to do "anything" might exceed parental ability or willingness. Parents must be prepared to recognize that help it isn't always wanted or valuable.

Serious Problems Can Be Encountered With Adolescents

In this section, I describe several of the more serious problems adolescents can encounter. It is not my intention to describe all of the horrible hypotheticals of adolescence. Most of the things that can go wrong can be worked through with an understanding of the process through which adolescents work to become adults. An understanding of the process of adolescence and some ability to tolerate ambiguity will help parents endure the transformation of their child through adolescence and on toward adulthood.

Depression and Suicide

Today suicide is the second leading cause of death for the adolescent and is exceeded only by accidents. Over the last 50 years, the life expectancy for all ages has appreciably lengthened except for that of the adolescent. For the adolescent, suicide rates quadrupled between 1950 and 1988 according to the Centers for Disease Control (1991). These are frightening numbers and represent a sad loss for society.

Nothing is more tragic and devastating for parents than the suicide of their child. There is almost always overwhelming guilt following such a death. It is human to seek answers to questions such as, "What did we do wrong?" and "What could we have done to prevent it?" Many children who end their life have given some sort of advance hint concerning their intentions, even though veiled and ill-defined. However, for others, it is an impulsive and unplanned act.

Some adolescents feel inadequate to cope with the challenges that come in the teenage years. In their self-evaluation, they might see a reprehensible self or merely come to the conclusion that they are worthless. I recall one adolescent girl who declared, "Of all the people in this entire universe that I might have become, I'd rather not have been me." Sometimes the feelings of despondency are so painful that an adolescent might try to substitute other affects, such as anger and fright.

The vast majority of adolescents do not kill themselves. One important consideration for parents is not hysterical panic but the recognition of the fact that although the majority of young people transact adolescence without killing themselves, the transaction is difficult, scary, and painful. Another consideration is that with the understanding and support of at least one parent, the adolescent can manage the process quite well.

Distinguishing real suicide threats from suicidal jargon.
Not all depressed adolescents seek suicide either. Some contemplate suicide, but never act on their impulse. Alternatively, they might engage in some other outrageous behavior that is simply a cry for help. Parents frequently hear, "I wish I were dead" from children

who are frustrated, angry, or hurt but who have absolutely no intention of ending their lives at all.

Some do more than threaten. Some put the threat into an action designed to express their feelings when words fail them. The term *suicide gesture* is sometimes applied to such actions but is, I believe, a risky concept in that it implies that the attempt does not need a serious response. Even suicide gestures need a prompt and clearly enunciated response, especially with children. They can be a red flag pointing to a serious, underlying problem, as in the following example:

> Donnie, a 15-year-old boy of borderline intellect, tried to kill himself, only to be found by his parents in a semiconscious state. He explained his despair with these words: "I'm going to fail at school again this year. My parents and my teachers have told me over and over that I have to graduate from high school and get a good education if I'm going to become somebody. No matter how hard I try, I can't make it! I guess I'll be a nobody!" His parents, teacher, and I benefited from his painful words. We concluded that, no matter how important a good education might be, its absence ought not call for ending a child's life.

Such acts carry with them hidden statements that must be understood. The very act suggests that the individual feels incapable of putting his or her desperation into words or fears that the words will not be understood. The suicide attempt can be a child's way of asking someone to stop doing something he or she is doing or to start doing something he or she is not doing. The other message is a plea for someone to care. Although it is not unheard of, young children are less inclined toward suicide than are adolescents. Adolescents are more likely to have access to the means of suicide than are younger children. Repeated attempts should be taken very seriously, as the law of averages will eventually catch up, or miscalculation may lead to death by misadventure.

Distinguishing sadness from depression.   Sadness is a condition of humankind, and the adolescent knows its taste. Depression is not the same as sadness. All people have occasional sadness, usually for apparent reasons. They have good days and bad days, but they shouldn't have bad days day in and day out.

Depression can be a consequence of the loss of something critically important in an adolescent's life or it might come "out of the blue," seemingly for no apparent reason. Depressive illnesses can lead to death. But depression can be treated. Antidepressant medications are effective in adolescents as well as adults. Some depressive illnesses carry a strong hereditary link. An adolescent can become depressed even though his or her life is seemingly going well otherwise. What makes depressive illnesses difficult to manage is the misunderstanding that surrounds them. Because depression is similar to sadness, it can go untreated unnecessarily. Urging depressed adolescents to "snap out of it" will do no good. They can't! They didn't "snap into it" in the first place, and urging them to snap out of it runs the risk of their believing that they can and should. Then, when they try to "snap out of it," they discover they can't escape their depressive feelings, and then feel worse.

Abuse

It helps to grow up in a highly competent family. But even there, things can go wrong. And when things go wrong, it is only human to begin casting about as to who the villain is. Often parents are the first ones that children blame for their problems; it has become a common practice to seek the roots of all adult problems in a childhood marred by "dysfunctional" parents. Parents who were themselves abused as children would seem more likely to be abusive. And yet, some who have endured unspeakable abuse become loving and protective parents.

Without a doubt, painful childhood experiences can have serious repercussions in adulthood. Sexual abuse, physical abuse, and emotional abuse are going to inflict not only physical bruises, but also psychological wounds, during both childhood and adulthood. Once they reach adolescence, children who have been abused might run away from home or begin to strike back, as in the following example:

Tommy was a bright 17-year-old boy who worked hard in school and made good grades. He had few friends. He would bring no one home with him. Tommy's father beat his mother and had beaten her even while she was carrying Tommy. Once Tommy was born, his father abused him and his mother continually. At age 17, Tommy ended the abuse when he shot and killed his father while defending his mother. He was set "free" by the legal system in that he wasn't sent to jail, but children who kill a parent usually don't do well in life, regardless of the circumstances.

Neglect

An even greater disservice can come in the form of neglect, for here a child is ignored as if he or she did not even exist. Perhaps never deprived of worldly goods or nutritional necessity, a child can experience a neglect of nurture, which leads to a poverty of self-worth. Never struck, never cursed, never abused—never noticed—a child might wonder if he or she exists in the eyes and hearts of those who are supposed to care for and about him or her. The following case example describes a child who had been treated in this way:

Jeremiah was age 17 when I first saw him. He was one of four children born to his natural parents, who were divorced, but the only one of those four of whom his father had custody. The father had remarried. He lived in his father's house with the new wife and her two children. Jeremiah was never close to anyone and felt he was the "odd man out" in his original family and in his father's new family.

Jeremiah had been referred to me by his school counselor because of poor grades. She had also detected in Jeremiah's affect a pervading sense of despair coupled with an aura of hopelessness, something that she felt might lead to suicide, although Jeremiah had made no overt attempts to take his life. He was also a loner at school.

When Jeremiah came to my office, he wore outrageous clothes that were only slightly less noticeable than his hair. A 3-inch band of almost day-glo orange hair stood at spiked attention from his forehead to the back of his skull, surrounded by a gleaming and freshly shaved scalp. His clothing was only slightly more conservative but clean. He responded positively to my questions and seemed eager for my acceptance. By the end of the hour, he could stand it no longer and asked me why I hadn't commented on his attire. When I asked, "Am I supposed to?" he shrugged and said "Everyone else does. If I didn't dress this way, no one would ever notice me!"

In her poem "A Choice of Weapons," McGinley (1954) describes the hurt that comes from being unnoticed.

Sticks and Stones are hard on bones.
Aimed with angry art,
Words can sting
like anything.
But silence breaks
the heart.

Although it is a poor consolation, the child who is abused at least has his or her existence validated.

Anorexia Nervosa and Bulimia Nervosa

Adolescent dysfunction can take many forms. Two of the most life-threatening and stubborn disorders are anorexia nervosa and bulimia nervosa. Adolescent girls are most likely to manifest these illnesses, although they occasionally occur in boys. They might present as a gorging of food, an absolute rejection of food, or a bedeviling combination thereof. These adolescents might gorge themselves, induce vomiting, and gorge again. They will exercise outrageously, and in secret if necessary, in order to avoid what they perceive as fatness. They will diet to a point of severe malnutrition while insisting that they need to lose weight. Some die. The presenting symptoms of these illnesses justifiably frighten parents. The central symptom of starvation is so compelling it cannot be ignored.

These disorders demand skilled treatment. Historically, treatment has focused on restoring body weight. However, effective treatment must go beyond merely combating the central symptom. With enough coercion, body weight can be restored even against the patient's wishes. To do so requires absolute control of the patient's life by the treatment personnel. It requires constant observation of each and every moment of the child's existence, even during sleep. Sure enough, the patient gains enough weight to be discharged from the hospital. And then what happens? The patient slips back to square one, as in the following case example:

> Francie began "dieting" when she was age 13. Her parents thought nothing of it at first as many adolescents worry about their bodies, even when the body is not a source of worry for anyone else. Soon the parents realized that all was not well. When they were unable to interrupt what they saw as self-starvation, they sought professional help. Francie was admitted to a hospital and soon regained the lost weight. She was discharged. Again, she went on a diet, secretly at first, and then openly. She was readmitted to the hospital, again looking like "skin and bones." Sure enough, she again renourished herself and was again discharged after several weeks.
>
> Eventually, Francie landed back in the hospital having once again lost a significant portion of her body weight. This time her physician was not easily persuaded that her problem would be solved with just adequate weight gain. He promptly referred her to me and recommended long-term care.
>
> Francie and her parents worked very hard during her stay in the hospital. Francie's underlying problem—depression—was diagnosed and treated. Like all adolescents, she was struggling with the conflictual issues of adolescence, but the process was obscured by the self-starvation. She had felt out of control of her life and had sought to impose a sense of self-control through her rigid dieting. It was a very maladaptive solution, but one that left her feeling in control. During her previous hospitalizations, her physician had had to take control of her life away from her and force her to gain weight in order to save her life. This course of action ultimately led to a repetition of maladaptive behavior. During her long-term hospitalization, Francie was able to gain an understanding of the underlying struggles and the treatment of her depression. She learned more adaptive ways to manage her life. Her parents persisted throughout a long battle for the life of their child; it was hard work for everyone involved.

Academic Dysfunction

One of the more troubling ways in which things can go wrong lies in the area of the adolescent's schoolwork. Although this topic doesn't involve a pathological illness, it does generate an enormous amount of anxiety for both parents and child. In fact, academic dysfunction might be more properly considered in the chapter on risk-taking behavior because it can have serious implications for the adolescent's future.

Poor performance and poor self-esteem are linked. A young child enters school where he or she is expected to learn new things and to master tasks appropriate to age and intellectual capacity. It is the child's first job. It is where he or she learns how to be industrious and to reap the rewards of success. Based upon his or her capacity to learn and upon the responses received from those who care, the child comes to value industry with its sense of competence or comes through the experience with a pervading sense of inferiority. School becomes not only a source of knowledge about the world but also a place where the child begins to formulate a view of self and how he or she fits into that world.

The child who has difficulty in acquiring knowledge is at risk in the formulation of self-esteem. Each child's individual capacity must be understood, so that reasonable expectations can be designed that are appropriate to that child's ability. Children who know the love and acceptance of parents and families will not lack self-esteem.

Poor academic performance is a transient symptom of normal adolescent struggles. Of all the adolescents I treated, almost all of them were having some sort of academic difficulty. A few of these adolescents made excellent grades but were nonetheless desperately ill. Some of them had withdrawn all effort, energy, and interest from the other parts of their lives and piled it all on academics.

Even the healthy, well-adjusted child might show evidence of academic loss at the onset of adolescence. Adolescence is a time of reordering, and, as physical, emotional, and social aspects of life surge, there is at least a temporary shifting of interests. But most adolescents recover their posture and take up where they left off in being responsible about their schoolwork.

Adolescents balk at parental control over their schoolwork. Many forces at work can complicate school issues. Because of the underlying control issues, parents and adolescents frequently come to confrontations. As cited in an earlier chapter, parents can become overly involved in their child's schoolwork and not fully realize that they might be making matters worse. Anther example of how this comes into play follows.

> Kent wasn't all that bright, but he was perfectly capable of passing his schoolwork. "I have to supervise his schoolwork constantly," his mother complained to me. "Every day I check his homework and see to it that he studies. He barely passes. I consult with his teachers. They say he could do better and that I should leave it up to him. Of course I worry about his schoolwork, because he never does. So far this year, we are passing all subjects." It must have been the look on my face that caused her to pause, recall her use of the word "we," and then blush. "Well, I mean he is passing. . . . I mean. . . . Well, I suppose I should say we. Perhaps I should have said I am passing all subjects." What a comfort it must have been to Kent to know that someone was actively engaged in worrying about his schoolwork!
>
> Kent's mother was an accomplished musician. She was highly intelligent, poised, and socially popular. She was an excellent athlete and a successful businesswoman. In Kent's eyes, she was powerful in so many ways. As he compared himself with her, he came off poorly in his own view.
>
> At some level, Kent's mother understood that it was Kent's responsibility to see to his schoolwork, but try as she might, she was unable to stop lecturing and cajoling him into doing the work. "I keep thinking that if I can say it one more time, or if I say it the right way, I'll somehow get through to him," she confessed. She was making herculean efforts to bolster her son's efforts but succeeded only in causing him to see himself as weak. In his view, his mother could do anything. But, in a hidden part of Kent's mind, there was some sort of consolation. In one small facet of his life, he was so powerful that he could figuratively bring her to

her knees. She could do anything except "make" him take over the worrying about his schoolwork.

With a great deal of help, Kent's mother renounced her role of being responsible for her son's acquisition of an education. With my help, she said to her son, "Kent, I want you to understand that I will no longer be responsible for your passing at school. No more pleading. No more bribing. No more threatening. It's up to you. If you fail, it's your fault. But if you pass, all of the credit will be yours."

Many parents face this challenge and have considerable difficulty extracting themselves. They are held hostage by the anxiety that swirls around relinquishing the role of the enforcer.

The average adolescent possesses a normal intellect. Children with an average IQ should be able to complete a high school education and even college, if so desired. "How do I motivate my child to make better grades?" has been a popular question asked by many of my patients' parents. It is always difficult to motivate oneself to do those things that one is not eager to do. Motivate others? That's very difficult. It's a good bit easier to demotivate. Parents do so by implying that they will be responsible for somehow providing the stimulus to see to it that their child does well at school or at work. What they might do instead is direct their child's attention to the objects of their responsibility.

Drug Use, Abuse, and Addiction

Drug use and abuse is discussed in Chapter 6 within the context of adolescents forming their self-identity. However, because drug use can be one of the major problems encountered by adolescents, I recapitulate some of the points here. I would like to note that when I speak of drugs, I am also referring to alcohol when used in excess.

Adolescents turn to drugs for two primary reasons. The first reason is that drugs and alcohol bring relief from psychological pain, such as that experienced when an adolescent feels especially conflicted as a result of the changes occurring within himself or herself, or when an adolescent is troubled in his or her home life. Second, adolescents may use drugs as a consequence of becoming involved in a peer group that uses drugs. The adolescent's main reason for turning to that peer group could be that he or she was rejected by the peer group of his or her choice. In a family troubled by teenage drug abuse, parents can refer to a useful resource: *Getting Tough on Gateway Drugs: A Guide for the Family* (DuPont 1984).

There is a difference between drug use, drug abuse, and addiction. With some drugs, use will become abuse. Some drugs have an almost irresistibly addictive quality, whereas still others do not necessarily lead to addiction. Some drugs are not addictive but, nevertheless, are harmful and even fatal.

The *Diagnostic and Statistical Manual of Mental Disorders, Fourth Edition* (DSM-IV) published by the American Psychiatric Association (1994) describes the principal disorders of drug use under the heading of substance-related disorders and points out that a wide variety of substances can result in what are designated as substance use disorders. Those disorders are substance abuse and substance dependence.

Substance abuse is defined as a maladaptive pattern of substance use leading to clinically significant distress, as manifested by one or more of the following during a 12-month period:

+ Recurrent use resulting in a failure to fulfill major role obligations at work, school, or home
+ Recurrent use in physically hazardous situations (e.g., driving, operating machinery)
+ Recurrent substance-related legal problems
+ Continued use despite persistent social or interpersonal problems caused by the substance use

Substance dependence results in symptoms that involve not only behavioral manifestations but also cognitive symptoms (such as memory deficit, disorientation, and language disturbances) and physiological symptoms. And the diagnosis of dependence indicates that the individual continues to use the substance despite all of the substance-related problems. The compulsive use of a substance is one of the hallmarks of substance dependence. When the individual shows not only compulsive use but also shows evidence of a need for increasing dosage (tolerance) and begins to experience unpleasant symptoms when attempting to reduce dosage (withdrawal), then the diagnosis of substance dependence with physiological dependence should be made. The latter is what is commonly called addiction.

Habitual use is different from addiction. The difference lies in not only the drug's capacity to addict but also the individual's capacity to resist. Although one might get into the habit of using a particular drug, that does not constitute addiction. Some drugs can be resisted. Others cannot. Some authorities in the field suggest that certain drugs aren't "all that bad" and might not do any damage. I have seen no studies that indicate that any of the "recreational" drugs in any way enhance the health and development of adolescents.

Conclusion

It is important to know that the vast majority of adolescents make the journey to adulthood without serious disorder in their lives. Do they accomplish this without anxiety, pain, or disappointment? Of course not. The vast majority of families are effective in providing a healthy environment in which children and adults can and do grow. Dysfunctional is a descriptive too glibly applied. Even competent families experience anxiety, pain, and disappointment as they move through their life cycle. Death, divorce, and deprivation make family life a struggle, but they don't necessarily prevent the mission of the family. I've seen some adolescents who have lost at least one parent and endured considerable deprivation, but who nonetheless turned out well and without psychiatric sequelae. And I've seen children with major psychiatric disorders come out of loving families.

When serious problems do arise, parents should seek the opportunities that accompany those crises to become more effective parents and subsequently more effective spouses. If parents can extend an attitude of inquiry and understanding to the problems in their lives, they will live more effective lives. No one wants things to go wrong. No one wants problems. But there are many golden opportunities walking around disguised as problems. Each problem contains the seed for its solution. Each problem in human relations can yield the opportunity for growth.

Late Adolescence

FEIFFER®

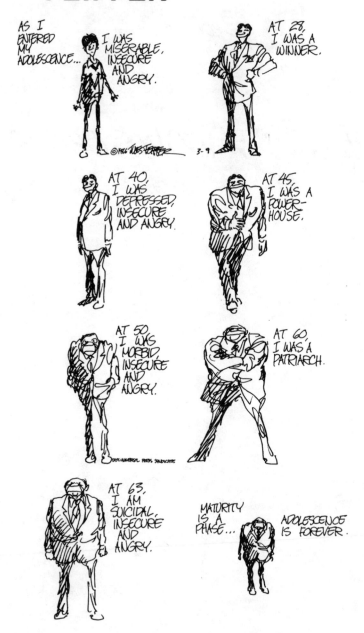

Chapter 10

Transition Into Adulthood

~~~~~~

*E*ventually adolescence is over. Around age 18 or 19, children begin to take on more and more adult status. Emancipation is not yet total, but it is well on the way. Few 18-year-old adolescents have reached a position of self-support sufficient to allow more than a moderate degree of autonomy. Financial independence eludes all but a few adolescents and, until such has been acquired, emancipation and autonomy cannot be complete. But there are degrees and stages of each that are appropriate and attainable during late adolescence and early adulthood.

Much of the psychological work of adolescence has been fulfilled by age 18. The sociological growth has progressed so that an 18- or 19-year-old individual is able to initiate and carry through new relationships with some degree of skill and comfort. It is a time of increased socializing, with some lengthening of the term of relationships. The completion of secondary education permits the beginning of a career in either the workplace or through further education and training. Although not yet fully mature, the young adult is ready for a more independent life and begins to function outside of the family in pursuit of increasing autonomy. Even when the young adult remains in the parental home, the relationship with his or her parents begins to define itself further. Parents can look forward to a reconnecting with their offspring in what begins to be a more gratifying relationship.

Leaving Home

Although economic factors bear on the young adult's ability to leave the parental home, some adolescents remain there for other reasons.

Single-Parent Homes

Single-parent homes might retain children later in life than do dual-parent homes. One reason for this could be that single-parent homes often have more constrained economic circumstances, thus making it more difficult for the single parent to assist a young adult in setting up an independent living situation. Guilt about abandoning the single parent might also prompt some young people to stay and take care of the parent. Much depends upon the intactness of the remaining parent and whether the relationship is one of need fulfillment.

Most single-parent homes are healthy and productive. Single-parent homes can move children toward autonomy and independence despite an absent parent. Indeed, a single-parent home can be more functional and healthier than a two-parent home if the latter is riven by dissension, distrust, and disloyalty.

Dual-Parent Homes

It does not necessarily follow that a dual-parent home is healthier or easier to leave than a single-parent home. As stated earlier, the most important contribution parents can make to the psychological health of their children is that they be able to meet each other's needs as a husband and wife. For example, when one parent reaches across the generational boundary and involves himself or herself in a need-fulfilling relationship with one or more of the children, the relationship then becomes a disabling one for both the parent and child. If one's concept of one's value and worth are inextricably bound in a need-fulfilling relationship, the loss of the relationship results in a loss of self-esteem and personal worthiness.

It is easier to leave home when one's parents have demonstrated an ability and willingness to take care of each other. There is comfort in knowing that the parental home remains intact and functional.

However, do not discount the fact that a young adult may choose to leave home precisely because it is an unhappy home.

Staying Home, But Leaving Adolescence

When a young adult must remain under the parental roof for economic reasons, it is still possible—indeed, it is necessary—for that young adult to move beyond adolescence. Both the young adult and his or her parent(s) can avoid his or her fixation in an adolescent mode. This hinges upon clear communication and an understanding of the underlying forces at work. Parents must ask themselves what psychological tasks the child must now accomplish, whether in the arena of home, school, or employment.

Erikson (1950) offered a readily understandable view of developmental issues through his description of the eight stages of human development. He postulated these stages as psychosocial tasks that had to be mastered. His concept is only one of many others, but it is easily understood and offers a measuring stick by which one might gauge an individual's growth.

Erikson postulates these stages as one outcome versus its opposite. For example, during the first 18 months of life, a child learns to either trust or mistrust his or her environment and its willingness to meet his or her basic needs. The outcome of this issue will do much to move the child forward in a trusting exploration of his or her life or possibly taint his or her view of the environment. Subsequent stages provide the child with the opportunities to develop autonomy versus shame and doubt, initiative versus guilt, and industry versus inferiority. During adolescence, Erikson postulates the challenge as identity versus role confusion. Once this task has been mastered, either adolescents have successfully consolidated their sense of identity and leave adolescence with a sense of who they are or else they leave adolescence in confusion about their role. And so, on to adulthood.

Indeed, each of the tasks of psychological growth has a time for its development. Pursuit of independence and autonomy is a task of adolescence and is appropriate at that time. Such a pursuit during childhood not only would fail but would have harmful consequences for the child's physical and emotional well-being. Society has learned that. It has withheld its approval of independence and autonomy until late adolescence and early adulthood, so that it will have beneficial rather than destructive consequences. Moreover, Judeo-Christian and Western culture has withheld its approval of early adolescent sexuality not only on a basis of moral issues but also on the incompleteness of psychological as well as social preparation.

True Intimacy and Adulthood

Early adulthood brings with it the prospect of seeking and finding a mate. Having reached a critical point in the process of becoming, each person seeks another who has similarly reached this critical point. Here begins a bringing together of two separate processes—each person is in the process of becoming a fully developed adult, and each will influence the other and be influenced in turn. At this point in life the individual develops a sense of being able to commit himself or herself to someone or something else.

Erikson defined the primary challenge of early adulthood as intimacy versus isolation. By developing a capacity for intimacy, a young adult can commit himself or herself to another human being in a mutually rewarding relationship. Failure to find this intimacy can lead to a sense of aloneness, distance, and separateness.

Whether this main challenge of adulthood can be met successfully depends upon whether the individual has mastered the challenges in the preceding stages of life. It will depend upon the individual's basic capacity for trust, sense of self-esteem, ability to explore the environment of places and people, sense of competence, sense of identity, and, above all, sense of being worthy of receiving another human being's love. Success in these areas will have been predicated on the type of support a person has received from his or her family throughout life: how well the family has been able to sustain each member through times of adversity, how each member feels about the others, and how each member feels about himself or herself. If an individual has reached this stage of life with an adequate resolution of all of those previous difficulties, chances for a successful outcome are good. If he or she has come to view other human beings with a basic mistrust, he or she will have learned to be suspicious of others, to expect betrayal, and to experience all efforts of gratification from the environment as being thwarted. Success or failure in the challenge to find intimacy will likewise influence the remaining challenges that a person comes to face.

For many young adults, the work of this psychological challenge will take place in the marriage. The establishment of a capacity for intimacy then becomes a joint task as well as two individual tasks. Each brings to the marriage and to the pursuit of intimacy his or her strengths and weaknesses. In this challenge, each person is exposed to his or her own process of becoming and that of another. In some ways, these two processes now become one. Or, perhaps three, because not only are we becoming who we are to be as individuals but also as a couple and as a family.

Finding the Appropriate Degree of Intimacy

Although the attainment of true intimacy is the antithesis of isolation, it should not suggest a loss of separateness and privacy. Even though a mastery of true intimacy brings the joy of closeness, there are limits of intimacy for each person. Early in adulthood the pursuit of intimacy leads toward the joining of two lives in marriage. Levinson (1978) labeled the early and mid-20s, when most first marriages occur, as *provisional adulthood,* thereby implying a process of evolving either toward a steady state or toward a regression. It is in these years that one's life work begins as well as the finding of a mate. Learning how to work and how to love become critical tasks for young adulthood.

Because each person comes to this task with different life experiences, different egos, and different capacities, the amount of intimacy desired is going to be different for each. Blaine (1962) suggested that newborns begin life with differing capacities for giving and receiving closeness, and described a continuum of receptivity, with huggers at one end and kickers at the other. Within the same family, one sees children who seek and accept the demonstration of affection from adults, whereas others shun it.

Children who observe sterile interactions between parents are subject to learning such behavior in their interactions with others. Children who discover the joy of having a chum of the same gender during their preadolescence and early adolescence have begun laying the foundation for the mastery of true intimacy with a member of the opposite gender later in young adulthood. True intimacy evolves from a willingness to share thoughts and feelings in a growing state of trust with another human being. It is during the verbal exchanges with a chum that we experience a relationship that is helpful in practicing a kind of closeness. A major benefit that comes from such a relationship is the realization that we are not all that different from our fellow human beings.

A close relationship with a member of the same gender also helps an individual to understand himself or herself and enhances his or her sense of what it means to be a man or to be a woman. The closeness of the relationship can be a source of anxiety if one has been taught that all feelings of tenderness and affection will lead to a sexual encounter. In the adolescent, and again in the young adult, feelings of affection for a member of the same gender can be misunderstood as homosexuality.

In addition, the young adult who has done the work of adolescence will find himself or herself better prepared for the pursuit of true intimacy. Completion of the work of adolescence should bring one to a new relationship with parents and other adults.

Spousehood Grows Through True Intimacy

The environment in which children grow best is one that is also conducive to adult growth. Spousehood grows through the pursuit of true intimacy. Achieving true intimacy is a consequence of revelation of oneself—a revelation of one's needs, one's hopes, and one's dreams. Out of these revelations comes a growing sense of trust and a growing sense of one's worth to each other. Through these experiences, the young wife and the young husband come to know each other's needs. Meeting each other's needs as a man and woman, as a husband and wife, and as a father and mother demonstrates to children the wondrous ways in which two human beings live together and care for each other. To the extent that a husband

and wife are able to achieve true intimacy with each other, the relationship will grow.

Commitment: Essential to Fulfillment in Life

Both occupation and marriage can lead to creativity and fulfillment. Producing a product or rendering a service allows one to be creative in one's work. Successfully finding a mate can also lead to creativity, such as the creation of another human being or the creation of a productive and fulfilling life. Central to these tasks is the capacity for commitment. The young adult who has attained a degree of physical health, coupled with intact and stable psychological health, comes to adulthood well equipped to make a commitment to another human being in a loving and supportive relationship.

True Intimacy and Accountability

However, commitment is not required in order to have sexual intercourse; it requires little in the way of personal investment and personal knowledge of each other. It can be, and frequently is, carried out by strangers who do not even know each other's name. Sexual intercourse can be one of the routes to growth and fulfillment in the lives of the partners—if it is part of a loving relationship that embraces commitment, loyalty, selflessness, and mutual respect.

Possessed of reproductive capacity, the young adult now moves away from isolation toward true intimacy with another, generativity, and parenthood. Society seeks a commitment between these potential parents as a means of promising commitment to and accountability for the offspring of their union. Simons (1985) defined true intimacy well:

> The capacity for true intimacy requires an integration of both love and sexual desire. It is free from excessive idealization as well as contemptuous hatred of the other person. And it rests on a secure sense of one's own self and one's own boundaries. Sexual

desire, orgasmic fulfillment and commitment to another do not pose any threat of personal dissolution. Two people can give themselves to each other and at the same time be enriched by the giving, not depleted. The identity of each becomes even further consolidated and expanded through their intimacy, not fragmented nor diminished. (p. 445)

Again, Simons (1985) cited a profound truth, ascribed to Tolstoy: "One can live magnificently in this world, if one knows how to work and how to love, to work for the person one loves, and to love one's work."

Productive Employment and Productive Relationships

Although people are not necessarily expected to remain in their first job, there is an expectation that they will remain in their first marriage. Because there is not an expectation of remaining in the relationship of our first choice, a kind of social trial and error is permitted. For both work and love, early adulthood provides time to discover how to do work and how to build a relationship. With an understanding of the requirements of productive employment, we will find a particular job to which we can give commitment. With an understanding of the requirements of a productive relationship, we will find a particular person to whom we can give commitment.

Earning Trust

The pursuit of true intimacy is a process of discovery. It requires a revelation of oneself to oneself as well as to another person. Such a pursuit requires a willingness to begin a process of growing trust. Most new relationships begin with very few reasons for trusting but also with very few reasons for not trusting each other. Lasting trust in a new relationship must be earned slowly.

Marriage

People bring to marriage certain expectations and certain unspoken assumptions. Often those expectations are fantastical, based on assumptions that will later be discovered to be different from the assumptions of one's chosen mate.

If the marriage is entered into with overwhelming expectations, it will fail. The young adult who approaches marriage as a substitute for other profound psychological needs might find gratification initially and disillusionment later. The joy that comes from being loved will not last unless returned. Romantic fantasies about love and marriage will not endure the stress and strains of everyday living. The romantic view of love casts the marital partner in the role of nurturer and grantor of unrealistic expectations and fails to see the partner as a person. The pursuit of true intimacy leads over pathways that help each partner see the other as a person in his or her own individuality but also helps each grow as individuals. Knowing each partner as a person helps each meet the other's needs.

Not all individuals arrive in young adulthood unscathed and unscarred. Because each brings invisible wounds to the state of matrimony, marriage has been described as an attempt at healing. Successful marriages bring the kind of personal experiences that can promote growth. Many minor wounds are thus healed in the give and take of living in a close relationship, if that alliance is blessed by clear and open communication in a setting of love, tolerance, and growing trust.

Parenthood and Creativity

Although the pursuit of true intimacy begins in young adulthood, the search extends into mid-life and even later. For some it remains ever beyond reach. But adulthood brings more than a search for true intimacy. Coupled with such a task is nature's principal injunction: reproduce, create. In exchange for these efforts lies the potential for growth and fulfillment of yet another of Erikson's (1950) psychological challenges: generativity versus stagnation. Many attain fulfillment of their creative urges through great works of art, literature, or music. For most, those urges bring forth children. Sadly, some of those children are brought forth by those who are not yet ready for such responsibility.

Parenthood offers the opportunity to be creative by producing new members of society. People have children for a variety of reasons, one of which is a sense of continuity. That sense provides them with a connection to the ensuing generation. Beyond the pursuit of true intimacy Erikson saw the challenge of adulthood as generativity, not only in creating children, but also in becoming the nurturers and mentors for the next generation. A sense of generativity and productivity in one's life and one's work adds to one's sense of fulfillment and growth.

Even good marriages between compatible and emotionally stable people are going to feel the challenges that come from the introduction of a newborn. Some of the attention given to each other now must be diverted to, and invested in, parenthood. The context of the family is an excellent setting for not only the creation and bringing to autonomy of children, but also the stabilization and fulfillment of the parents.

It is during adolescence that parents begin to take on their challenge of becoming the mentors of the next generation. With an understanding of a mentor as a wise and trustful counselor, the successful parent begins to assume the role of consultant as he or she provides valuable advice in a setting of loving care. Much of character structure is formed by the time of adolescence. What the adolescent needs is a parent or parents who are at a point in their lives when they are becoming the wise and trusted counselors.

Parents of little children must be more than wise counselors and must take upon themselves the responsibility of diligent supervisors. Adolescents still need supervision, to a degree, but parents must begin to shift the responsibility of supervision more and more to the adolescent and begin to become the wise and trusted counselor for their delegate to the next generation.

Conclusion

And so older adolescents, their work of adolescence now done, become young adults in pursuit of true intimacy. Once a young adult achieves true intimacy with another, he or she becomes an adult capable of creativity and generativity. With the birth and development of their own child, these ex-adolescents now become the parents, soon to be awaiting the adolescence of their child. How sweetly doth nature bring about her rewards—and her revenge!

Parents of today's adolescents, take heart! Because eventually, it's all over. There is a life after children, with its challenge and reward. A wise man once declared, "The reason grandchildren and grandparents get along so well together is that they have a common enemy: the parents!"

True intimacy comes slowly. It is not available in an instantaneous form. It is a part of the process of becoming. The wondrous joy of a truly intimate relationship with another human being is the magnet that pulls us in the direction of growing trust and fulfillment. Although we select mates for various reasons, each of us seeks the other with hope and expectation. We hope to matter to someone. Each brings a life that has been influenced by those who brought about that life and by his or her ability to care for another.

Becoming Who One Was Meant to Be

Once the struggles of adolescence are completed, what comes next? Perhaps the most important psychological task of all: coming to terms with what a person has become. An adult must integrate all of the beliefs about himself or herself into a sense of who he or she has become. Erikson described the challenge in a clear and cogent choice: ego integrity versus despair. He defined *ego integrity* as "the acceptance of one's 'one and only' life cycle as something that had to be and that, by necessity, permitted of no substitutions" (Erikson 1950, p. 261).

For many, this self-evaluation begins in mid-life at about the time one's own children reach adolescence. The ferment of adolescent questioning and seeking triggers in the adolescent's parents a similar process of inquiry. Not only are the parents reminded of their past as they observe their adolescent, but they are also given a glimpse of their future. The adolescent's move toward an adult identity reminds the parents that they too are growing older. The adolescent's increasing sexuality contrasts with the gradual waning of sexuality of mid-life and later. The adolescent's increasing autonomy and independence find a different prospect in parents who are moving toward later life with decreasing independence. The adolescent's search for identity poses the question as to who he or she will become, whereas parents are beginning to seek an understanding of who they have become. The adolescent's and parents' searches exist in parallel, each influencing the other.

One's attempt to "see" what he or she has become is fed by a continuous stream of information from our environment and the people in that environment. However, this process is flawed by information that is unreliable. One's mind must continually seek out the information that is most wanted or needed—some may give negative feedback, which one may try to discount; others may give falsely positive feedback, knowing that one needs or wants to hear it. Depending upon how the person feels about himself or herself, he or she will selectively choose the information that is most wanted or needed, depending on how he or she feels about himself or herself. People stumble forward in life listening to one voice, then another, never quite certain about who they are or what they could be.

Coming to terms with one's own life does not happen spontaneously but rather is the result of psychological work—rooted in the care one received, and hence the trust one developed, in infancy—that is carried out over time in the context of living and interacting with family and friends. Fortunately, one's view of the environment and oneself can change. Corrective living experiences can and do intervene in the life of a child and can affect or even undo earlier negative experiences.

If one is going to come to terms with what one has become, he or she must lay claim to all of his or her existence—the good and the bad. Only that individual is primarily responsible for what he or she has become. Accepting this understanding leads to the discovery that one is in charge of what one is yet to be. As one grows, one also comes to terms with one's uniqueness. As one begins to assimilate an impression of who he or she is and is becoming, that person faces the challenge of personal discovery. He or she must not only begin a critical review of life so far, but must also make value judgments about the results so far.

It is with honesty, introspection, and objectivity that one begins to come to terms with life. This self-evaluation must also be approached with compassion. Sometimes it is easier to shrink from recognizing one's attractive qualities and unattractive qualities.

The successful resolution of this great challenge brings fulfillment of a life well lived and a sense of success. Psychological work is hard and sometimes painful.

Conclusion

~~~~~~

Adolescence is a small part of the wondrous human experience. One who attempts to understand adolescents without looking beyond the horizon will be viewing them only narrowly. It is appropriate to understand childhood as an important cross-section of a life to come. As parents, you are a revelation of what your adolescent's life will become, and you facilitate that by conducting your own life. Coming to know oneself and to know each other in a loving and accepting relationship is one of the essential pathways to fulfillment.

Parents are more likely to understand their adolescents if they understand the challenges they face. Adolescents are in a process of change, but that process does not end with the passage into adulthood. The ultimate goal of the maturing adolescent is not the acquisition of emancipation, independence, and autonomy, nor is it the establishment of a sense of identity—either gender or self. The psychosocial developmental destiny of the adolescent is beyond identity, through the attainment of true intimacy with another human being, on to generativity, and finally, to the fulfillment of integration of all aspects of being. Ultimately, each human being must come to terms with his or her self, finally, past, and future.

You, as parents, should take a step back and reflect on where you have been, where you are now, and where you are headed. Contemplate the process of adolescence and what it is doing to your child. Perhaps you already understand this process, but can you see what is happening to you? Not only is your child growing, but so are you. If you can understand the challenges your child now faces, you can help him or her grow. But there should be something in it for you as well. At adolescence, your child begins a departure from the safety and comfort of the family. That can be frightening for the child and frightening for you. But help your child leave, if you can. It's not the end.

One mother expressed this plea to all adolescents on behalf of parents: "Look, we are here, you need us, we are ready to help you. But in exchange, please give us a little attention." The poignancy of her plea was not missed. Although parents are available and ready to help, their pain comes from the fact that as adolescents approach adulthood, they need their parents less and less. "Give us a little attention" falls on otherwise distracted adolescent ears. Parents must begin to find that attention elsewhere. The more likely source lies within themselves and those with whom they have established intimate relationships.

There is something about surrendering parenthood that inflicts feelings of failure. If parents are to measure their success, they must use a worthy measuring stick. Ralph Waldo Emerson defined success in simple, but moving words:

> To laugh often and much; to
> win the respect of the
> intelligent people and the
> affection of children; to
> earn the appreciation of
> honest critics; to endure the
> betrayal of false friends; to appreciate
> beauty, to find the best in
> others; to leave the world a
> bit better, whether by a healthy
> child, a garden patch, or a
> redeemed social condition;
> to know even one life has
> breathed easier because
> you have lived. This is to
> have succeeded.

To share a life with another human being in a close and intimate and loving relationship is a wondrous experience. To have that experience lead to responsible parenthood, either through the creation of a child or by adoption, is to know an additional measure of joy. The struggle of ensuring the safety and fulfillment of that additional life can be daunting. Those who are still involved in the role of active parenthood should take hope and comfort in the knowledge gained from an understanding of the challenges that their adolescent faces. An understanding of the process of adolescence might bring to parents the answers to some of the questions posed at the outset of this book. Those questions concerned normal young people, not delinquent or psychopathic individuals, but those who live with us in our homes or nearby. But even with normal adolescents, life can be exciting and lively as their parents.

Having an insight into adolescent development and into their own development, parents will be better prepared to help their child become a fully functional adult, ready to accept a place of responsibility in society. An added benefit will be the considerable joy that comes from living in the daily give and take of that wonderful psychological support system known as the human family.

References

American Psychiatric Association: Diagnostic and Statistical Manual of Mental Disorders, 4th Edition. Washington, DC, American Psychiatric Association, 1994

Bailey JM, Pillard RC: A genetic study of male sexual orientation. Arch Gen Psychiatry 48:1089–1096, 1991

Blaine G: Patience and Fortitude. Boston, MA, Little, Brown, 1962

Cameron K: Diagnostic categories in child psychiatry. Br J Med Psychol 28:67–71, 1955

Centers for Disease Control: Attempted suicide among high school students—United States 1990. JAMA 266:1911–1912, 1991

Collange C: Today's adolescents, in International Annals of Adolescent Psychiatry, Vol 1. Edited by Esman A, Feinstein S, Lebovici S. Chicago, IL, University of Chicago Press, 1988, pp 1–4

Derdeyn A, Waters D: Parents and adolescents: empathy and the vicissitudes of development. Annals of Adolescent Psychiatry 5:175–185, 1977

DuPont RL Jr: Getting Tough on Gateway Drugs: A Guide for the Family. Washington, DC, American Psychiatric Press, 1984

Erikson EH: Identity vs. role diffusion, in Childhood and Society. New York, WW Norton, 1950, pp 261–263

Freud S: A General Introduction to Psycho-Analysis: A Course of Twenty-Eight Lectures Delivered at the University of Vienna. Translated by Riviere J. New York, Liveright Publishing, 1935

Grossman F, Beinashowitz J, Anderson K, et al: Risk and resilience in young adolescents. Journal of Youth and Adolescence 21:521–550, 1992

Josselyn I: Adolescence. New York, Harper & Row, 1971

Levinson D: The Seasons of a Man's Life. New York, Albert A Knopf, 1978

Lewis J: The impact of adolescent children on family systems, in Adolescent Psychiatry, Vol 13. Edited by Feinstein S, Esman A, Looney J, et al. Chicago, IL, University of Chicago Press, 1986, pp 29–43

Lewis JM, Beavers WR, Gossett JT, et al: No Single Thread: Psychologic Health in Family Systems. New York, Brunner/Mazel, 1976

McGinley P: A Choice of Weapons, in Times Three. Viking Press, 1954 (Originally appeared in New Yorker Magazine)

Offer D: The Psychological World of the Teenager. New York, Basic Books, 1969

Offer D, Offer J: Teenage to Young Manhood: A Psychological Study. New York, Basic Books, 1975

Offer D, Ostrow E, Howard K, et al: The Teenage World: Adolescents' Self-Image in Ten Countries. New York, Plenum, 1988

Offer D, Ostrow E, Howard K, et al: Adolescence: what is normal? Am J Dis Child 143:731–736, 1989

Orvin G: Intensive treatment of the adolescent and his family. Arch Gen Psychiatry 31:801–806, 1974

Piaget J: The Psychology of Intelligence. London, Routledge & Kegan Paul, 1950

Rand A: The Virtue of Selfishness. New York, Penguin Books, 1961

Simons R (ed): Understanding human behavior, in Health and Illness, 3rd Edition. Baltimore, MD, Williams & Wilkins, 1985, pp 445–450

Tolstoy L: Anna Karenina. London, Heinimann Publishers, 1901

Visher B, Visher J: Step-Families. New York, Brunner/Mazel, 1979

Index

~~~~~~

Page numbers printed in **boldface** *type refer to tables.*

Abstaining from sex, 118–119
Abstract thinking, 94–95
Abuse, 4, 151–152
Academic dysfunction, 155–157
    as control issue, 156–157
    poor self-esteem and, 155
    as transient symptom of
        normal adolescence,
        155–156
Academic performance, 63, 77–79,
    87–88, 127, 133–134
Accountability, 4, 55, 137
    intimacy and, 169–170
Addiction, 157–159
Advice giving, 146
Aggressivity, 85, 116
AIDS, 114
Alcohol use and abuse, 101–102,
    131–132, 157–159
Anger, 10, 46, 83
Anorexia nervosa, 153–154
Antidepressants, 151
Anxiety of adolescents, 43–44
Anxiety of parents, 84
Appearance of adolescent, 74, 83
Approval
    of adolescent by peers, 74,
        96–97

adolescents' beliefs about
    parents opinions of
    them, 98–100
adolescents' feeling of being
    loved, 84
parents' need for children's
    approval, 34
poor self-image and seeking
    approval elsewhere,
    100–102
withdrawal of parental
    approval, 60–61
Asking questions of adolescents,
    48–49
Authority of parents, 16
Autonomy of adolescents, 5–6
    as developmental task,
        165–166
    in late adolescence, 163
    parental reactions to
        emergence of, 29–32
    parental relationship and, 8

Behavior of adolescents
    constant changes in, 76–77
    criteria for interpretation of,
        86–88

Behavior of adolescents *(continued)*
    criteria for interpretation of
        adolescent who is having
            trouble in all areas, 88
        functioning in relation to
            friends, 88
        getting along with family,
            86–87
        performance on job, 87–88
    gender-specific, 108–110
    illogical, 133
    normal behaviors, 77–84, **78.**
        See also Normality in
        adolescents
    risk taking, 55, 125–137
    sexual, 105–122
    working with troubled
        adolescents, 89–91
Birth control, 112–114
Breast development, 106, 108
Bulimia nervosa, 153–154

Caregiving, 5, 25
Cause and effect, 127
Cautiousness of parents, 5–6, 30
Child abuse, 4, 151–152
Child custody hearings, 141
Child neglect, 152–153
Clumsiness, 106, 107
Commitment, 169–171
Communication, 37–52
    about sex, 112–113
    adolescents' difficulty in
        talking with adults, 45
    adolescents' expression of
        positive and negative
        feelings, 46–47, 82–83
    adolescents' initiation of,
        47–48
    as anxiety-producing
        experience for
        adolescents, 43–44
    asking how adolescent's life is
        going, 144–145
    asking questions, 48–49
    confidentiality of, 51
    confirming your
        understanding of
        adolescent, 41
    content of, 38
    in dysfunctional families, 20
    enhancing likelihood of
        adolescent confiding
        problems, 145–146
    gaining reassurance from
        adolescents, 47
    guidelines for, 33, 47–51
    in healthy families, 15
    to help prevent adolescents'
        risky behavior, 135
    hidden meanings in, 42–43,
        118
    honesty in, 48
    listening, 38–41, 44, 49–50
    loud, 45–46
    nature of, 38
    nonverbal, 41–42
    between parents, 51–52
    process of, 38
    of rules, 58
    by silence, 42
    teaching adolescents to
        disagree with respect,
        45–46
    words versus behavior, 50–51
Compassion, 69, 175
Competence of family, 15–22
    competent family, 17
    dysfunctional family, 17–22
    optimally competent family,
        15–17
Concrete thinking, 94
Condoms, 113, 114
Confidentiality, 51
Connectedness, 5, 6
Conscience, 82
Consequences
    of adolescents breaking rules,
        62–63

adolescents developing sense
of, 127
increased risk and, 55
of parents not relinquishing
all-powerful image, 27–28
Considerate behavior, 81
Constructive risks, 127–128
Contraception, 112–114
Control issues, 53–56. *See also*
Discipline; Limit setting;
Rules
in eating disorders, 153–154
increased difficulty in
controlling adolescents,
54–55
increased risk and
consequences for
adolescents, 55
reasons for adolescents'
resisting parental
control, 55–56
related to academic
dysfunction, 156–157
Creativity, 169, 171–172
Crime, 4, 55, 125
Criticism, 6
Crushes, 108
Curiosity, 127
"Cut-downs," 77

*D*ares, 129
Death, 4, 9, 109, 159
Decision-making skills, 147–148
Definition of family, 3–4
Demythologizing, 26–27
effect on parents, 29–32
long process of, 28
Depression, 31, 82, 87, 149–151
distinguishing from sadness,
150–151
suicide and, 149–150
treatment of, 151
Destructive risks, 128–129. *See
also* Risk-taking behavior

Developmental stages, 94–95, 165
Dieting, 153–154
Discipline, 33. *See also* Limit
setting; Rules
appropriateness of, 63–64
communication and, 50
guidelines for enforcing
limits, 61–64
self-discipline, 136
in stepfamilies, 13
withdrawal of parental
approval, 60–61
Disobedience, 66. *See also* Limit
setting; Rules
Disruption of family, 4, 9. *See also*
Structure of family
Divorce, 4, 9–11, 109, 159
adolescence as trigger for, 9
custody hearings and, 141
effects on children, 10, 142
personal growth after, 10
serious adolescent problems
related to, 141–143
Dress, 74, 83
Driving privileges, 63–64
Drug use and abuse, 4, 101–102,
125, 127, 129–132,
157–159
Dysfunctional family, 17–22, 159
genetic risks and, 19–20
inability to communicate
feelings in, 20
modern-day stresses and, 21–22
parental attitudes and beliefs
in, 18–19
parents engaging in
need-fulfilling
relationship in,
21, 31, 164
parents without self-esteem
and, 21
unhealthy environment and, 20

*E*ating disorders, 153–154
Eating patterns, 143

Ego development, 95–96, 100
Emancipation process, 28–29
Embarrassment, 106, 107
Emergency situations, 140
Emotional abuse, 151
Employment, 170
Encouraging adolescents, 5
Environment, unhealthy, 20
Erections, 106, 107
Erikson, E., 95, 165, 171, 173
Expression of feelings, 45–47,
    82–83. *See also*
    Communication
Extended family, 3–4

*F*amily as source of healing,
    90–91
Father-daughter relationship,
    120, 121
Father-son relationship, 26, 29,
    79–80, 109–110
Fear, 83
Financial independence, 163
"Finding" oneself, 93. *See also*
    Personal identity
Flexibility, 15
Food, 5
Foolish behavior, 129
Formal operations, 94–95
Freedom, 75
Friendships, 81–82, 88
    adolescent's functioning in
        relation to friends, 88
    of boys, 107
    of girls, 108
    parents as friends, 34
Fulfillment in life, 169–171

*G*angs, 125
Gender identity development,
    79–80, 108–111
    adolescent's need for same-
        gender model, 108–110
    homosexuality, 96, 110–111,
        168

Generativity versus stagnation,
    171
Genetic risks, 19–20
Gonorrhea, 114
Grandparenting, 173
Growth spurt, 107
Guidelines for effective parenting,
    32–35
    communicating with
        adolescents, 33, 47–51
    enforcing limits, 61–64
    preventing adolescents' risky
        behavior, 134–137
    setting limits, 57–60
Guilt, 82

*H*appy families, 3
Health care, 5
Homosexuality, 96, 110–111, 168
Honesty, 48, 68
Hormonal changes, 106–108
    in young females, 107–108
    in young males, 107
Housing, 5
Humor, 76–77

*I*dealism of adolescents, 50
Identity of adolescent, 93–103.
        See also Personal identity
Identity of family, 3
Ignoring adolescent, 152–153
Illogical behavior, 133
Immaturity, 66
Incest, 21, 120, 131
Inconsiderate behavior, 81
Individuality, 5
Industriousness, 68–69
Influence of parents, 70
Intelligence quotient, 77, 94, 157
Intimacy, 166–173. *See also* Sexual
        identity
    accountability and, 169–170
    definition of, 169–170

developing capacity for,
166–167
earning trust, 170
finding appropriate degree of,
167–168
versus isolation, 166, 167
spousehood growing through,
168–169
Irritability, 106, 107, 143
Isolation, 166, 167

*J*ealousy, 13, 81, 83
Judgment, 147–148
Justice, 69–70

*L*eadership of parents, 33
Learning by mistakes, 80
Leaving home, 164–165
in dual-parent homes,
164–165
in single-parent homes, 164
staying home but leaving
adolescence, 165–166
Lecturing of adolescent, 50
Lesbianism, 110
Limit setting, 53–70. *See also*
Discipline; Rules
adolescence as period of
increased responsibility,
54–56
increased difficulty in
controlling
adolescents, 54–55
increased risk and
increased
consequences, 55
reasons adolescents resist
parental control, 55–56
for adolescent who seems out
of control, 65–70
child's progress toward
adult functioning,
67–68

emotionally immature
adolescent, 66
evaluating child's qualities,
68–70
intensity of parental
efforts, 66–67
mentally ill adolescent, 66
parental influence, 70
unity of parents, 67
enforcing limits, 60–64
guidelines for, 61–64
withdrawal of parental
approval, 60–61
guidelines for making rules,
57–60
necessity for young children,
56–57
related to adolescent's future,
64–65
shifting to adolescent, 64–65
Listening, 38–41, 44, 49–50. *See
also* Communication
conveying interest by, 40
in order to understand,
39–40
with the third ear, 38–39
Loss, 32
Love, 34–35, 84
Lying, 68

*M*alnutrition, 153
Marriage, 6. *See also* Parental
relationship
true intimacy and, 167–169
in young adulthood, 170–171
Masturbation, 107
Media and sex, 111–112
Menstruation, 106, 107
Mental illness, 66, 125, 143–144
Mid-life challenges, 29–30, 173
Modeling, 7
of gender-specific behaviors,
108–110
of personal responsibility, 136

Moodiness, 76, 93, 143
Morality, 4
Mother-daughter relationship, 30,
    79–80, 108–110
Mother-son relationship,
    120–121
Motivation, 157

*N*eed-fulfilling relationships,
    21, 31, 164
Neglect, 152–153
Normality in adolescents, 73–91
    continual behavior changes,
        76–77
    definition of, 75
    determining when something
        is wrong, 86–88
    normal behaviors, 77–84, **78**
        appearance, 83
        being considerate, 81
        emotions felt and
            expressed, 82–83
        feeling loved, 84
        gender identification, 79–80
        learning by mistakes, 80
        loosening ties with family,
            81–82
        reaction to rules, 80–81
        remorse felt and shown, 82
        responsibility for
            schoolwork, 77–79
        tidiness and untidiness,
            83
        worrying the older
            generation, 84
    Offer studies of, 75–76
    parental reaction to, 84–85
    preadolescence and, 74–75
Nuclear family, 3–4

*O*ffer Self-Image Questionnaire,
    76
Omnipotence of adolescence,
    126

*P*arental attitudes and beliefs
    adolescents' beliefs about
        parents' opinions of
        them, 98–100
    avoiding "know-it-all"
        attitude, 147
    believing in their child,
        134–135
    in dysfunctional family, 18–19
    giving advice, 146
Parental cautiousness, 5–6
Parental need for children's
    approval, 34
Parental reactions to adolescent's
    emancipation, 29–32
    adjustment to diminishing
        role, 31–32
    adolescent's new
        independence, 30–31
    continuing role, 32
    first harbinger of change,
        29–30
Parental relationship, 4, 6–9
    caring about each other, 7–8
    characteristics of effective
        marriage, 6
    communication, 51–52
    in competent family, 17
    differences in child-rearing
        philosophies, 67
    divorce, 9–11
    effective parenting and, 6–7
    encouraging children's
        autonomy, 8
    incest and, 120, 131
    in optimally competent
        family, 15–17
    for problem solving, 8–9
    reevaluating personal growth, 8
    serious adolescent problems
        related to, 141
    within stepfamilies, 12–14
    taking time for oneself, 7, 22
Parental self-esteem, 21
Parenthood, 171–172

Parents Without Partners, 11

Peer approval, 74

Peer relationships, 81–82, 88
  adolescent's need for, 101
  drug- and alcohol-related peer
    groups, 101–102, 158
  of early adulthood, 170
  influence on development of
    personal identity, 96–97
  of late adolescence, 163
  transient influence of, 97

Perseverance, 69

Personal identity, 93–103, 165
  adolescents with poor
    self-image, 100–102
  developing powers of
    self-analysis, 94–96
  changing from concrete to
    abstract thinking,
    94–95
  using new skills to form
    self-identity, 95–96
  parental influence on
    development of, 97–100
  peer group influence on
    development of, 96–97
  social validation, 96–97
  transience of, 97

Physical needs of family
  members, 5

Piagetian stages of development,
  94–95

Poverty, 4

Power of parents, 25–32
  adolescent's demythologizing
    of, 26–27
    effect on parents, 29–32
    fears associated with, 27
    long process of, 28
  changing view of, 25–28
  consequences of not
    relinquishing
    all-powerful image,
    27–28
  sharing power, 15, 16

young children's projection
  of, 26

Preadolescence, 74–75, 94, 106, 107

Pregnant adolescent, 114–115, 125

Prepuberty, 106

Privileges of adolescents, 5, 32, 75
  driving, 63–64
  withdrawal as form of
    punishment, 62–64

Problems in adolescence, 139–159
  abuse, 151–152
  academic dysfunction,
    155–157
  actions before problems
    become serious, 144–148
  asking how adolescent's
    life is going, 144–145
  avoiding "know-it-all"
    attitude, 147
  being a good consultant,
    146–147
  creating atmosphere to
    enhance
    communication,
    145–146
  letting adolescent develop
    own judgment,
    147–148
  recognizing importance of
    adolescent's problem,
    147
  recognizing when help is
    wanted, 148
  anorexia nervosa and bulimia
    nervosa, 153–154
  depression and suicide,
    149–151
  drug use, abuse, and
    addiction, 101–102,
    129–132, 157–159
  due to psychiatric disorders,
    143–144
  gradual development of,
    140–141
  neglect, 152–153

Problems in adolescence
(continued)
parents trying to do their best
about, 139–140
reasons for development of,
139
related to divorce, 141–143
related to parents who are
unhappy together, 141
working with troubled
adolescents, 89–91
Problem-solving skills, 86, 141
letting adolescent develop for
self, 146–148
parental relationship for, 8–9
related to divorce, 10–11
for working with troubled
adolescents, 89–91
Protectiveness, 54–55, 90
Proverb interpretation, 94–95
Provisional adulthood, 167
Psychiatric disorders, 66, 125,
143–144
Psychological chaos of
adolescence, 73
Psychological growth, 100–101
becoming who one was
meant to be, 173–175
developmental tasks of,
165–166
after divorce, 10
within marriage, 8
of single parents, 12
Psychological impact of
adolescent sexual activity,
115–117
on females, 116–117
on males, 115–116
Puberty, 106
Punishment. See Discipline;
Limit setting

Quality time, 22
Questioning adolescents, 48–49

Rape, 125
Relationships of adolescent
with family, 86–87, 163
with parents, 120–121
with peers, 81–82, 88
Remorse, 82
Respect for others, 4, 16, 33–34, 66
teaching adolescents to
disagree with, 45–46
Respect for self, 136–137
Responsibility of adolescents,
5, 32
limit setting and increases in,
54–56
parental modeling and, 136
for schoolwork, 63, 77–79
self-responsibility, 33, 136–137
Responsibility to oneself, 7, 22
Right and wrong, 69–70, 82, 146
Risk-taking behavior, 55, 125–137
constructive risks, 127–128
destructive risks, 128–129
looking beyond, 129–132
parents' trouble in
understanding, 132–134
reasons for, 125–128
desire to move into
adulthood, 126–127
sense of omnipotence, 126
what parents can do to
prevent, 134–137
believe in their children,
134–135
help adolescents not need
to engage in risky
behavior, 135–137
Robbery, 125
Role confusion, 165
Role diffusion, 95
Roles of family, 4–9
developing parents'
personalities and their
relationship, 6–9
leading children toward
autonomy, 5–6

providing for physical needs
of family members, 5
Rules. *See also* Discipline; Limit
setting
adolescents' reaction to, 80–81
changing of, 60
clear statement of, 58
consequences of breaking,
62–63
consistency of, 59–60
content of, 57
enforcing of, 61–64
guidelines for making, 57–60
to provide safety, 59
purpose of, 57–58
shifting to adolescent, 64–65
testing of, 59
value of, 57

$\mathcal{S}$adness, 18, 83
distinguishing from
depression, 150–151
Safe sex, 114
Safety, 5
Schizophrenia, 144
Schoolwork. *See* Academic
dysfunction; Academic
performance
Self-analysis, 94–96
Self-discipline, 136
Self-esteem
of adolescents, 93–103. *See
also* Personal identity
of parents, 21
poor academic performance
and, 155
Self-evaluation, 8, 94–96, 173–175
Self-respect, 136–137
Self-responsibility, 33, 136–137
Sex education, 119
Sexual abuse, 151
Sexual development, 106–108
of boys, 107
of girls, 107–108

Sexual identity, 85, 105–122, 166.
See also Intimacy
changes in relationships with
parents, 120–121
early adolescent sexual
activity, 111–113
dangers of, 111, 113–115
encouraged by popular
media, 111–112
maturity enhances
sexuality, 117–118
mixed messages from
parents about, 112–113
psychological impact on
females, 116–117
psychological impact on
males, 115–116
forcing adolescent to abstain
from sex, 118–119
gender identity development,
108–111
hormonal changes, 106–108
marital relationship and
incest, 120
in new stepfamilies, 121–122
parents and their children's
sexuality, 119–120
Sexually transmitted diseases,
113–114, 125
Sibling rivalry, 81
in stepfamilies, 13
Single-parent families, 11–12
adolescent leaving home in,
164
challenges of, 11
parent acting as child's friend
in, 34
personal growth within, 12
psychological support for,
11–12
Sleeping patterns, 143
Smoking, 113, 126
Social problems, 4
Social validation, 96–97
Social withdrawal, 144

Starvation, 153
Stealing, 68
Stepfamilies, 12–14
    developing trust in, 12–13
    discipline in, 13
    opportunities provided by, 14
    rivalries in, 13
    sexuality and, 121–122
Strictness, 58, 90. *See also*
        Limit setting
Structure of family, 9–14
    changes after divorce, 9–11
    single-parent families, 11–12
    stepfamilies, 12–14
Substance abuse, 101–102, 125,
        127, 129–132, 157–159
    definitions related to, 158
Substance dependence, 158–159
Suicidal behavior, 125, 140, 143,
        149–151
    distinguishing real suicide
        threats from suicidal
        jargon, 149–150
    increases in, 149
    parental guilt about, 149
    repeated suicide attempts, 150
    suicide gestures, 150
Support system within family,
        3–4
Syphilis, 114

*T*asks of adolescence, 95
Tidiness, 83
Time for oneself, 7, 22
Time spent with children, 22
Transition into adulthood,
        163–175
    becoming who one was
        meant to be, 173–175
    changing relationship with
        family, 163
    commitment to employment
        and intimate
        relationship, 169–171

developing capacity for true
        intimacy, 166–167
    earning trust, 170
    financial independence, 163
    finding appropriate degree of
        intimacy, 167–168
    leaving home, 164–165
        dual-parent homes,
            164–165
        single-parent homes, 164
    marriage, 170–171
    parenthood and creativity,
        171–172
    spousehood growing through
        true intimacy, 168–169
    staying home but leaving
        adolescence, 165–166
Troubled adolescents
    criteria for interpreting
        behavior, 86–88
    mental illness, 66
    who seem out of control,
        65–70
    working with, 89–91
        family as source of healing,
            90–91
        looking to context of
            family, 89
        parental unity in
            approaching
            problems, 90
        searching for a solution, 89
Trust, 12–13, 165, 170
Truthfulness, 68
Turmoil of adolescence, 73

*U*nity of parents, 67, 90
Untidiness, 83

*V*alues, 4, 47, 112

*W*orking, 163
Worrying the older generation, 84